Biomedical Materials for Multi-functional Applications

Series Editors

Arnab Chanda, Centre for Biomedical Engineering, Indian Institute of Technology Delhi, New Delhi, Delhi, India

Sarabjeet Sidhu, Department of Mechanical Engineering, Sardar Beant Singh State University, Gurdaspur, Punjab, India

The series 'Biomedical Materials for Multi-functional Applications' is intended for the audience with an interest in biomaterials for various applications, including bio-implants, bio-instrumentation, biomechanics, and tissue engineering. The book titles under this series will bring different areas of biomedical engineering, bioengineering, materials science, mechanical engineering, and biosciences under one umbrella of biomedical materials. The books in this series will provide deep insights into the state-of-art of biomedical materials and deal with diverse and interdisciplinary aspects of biomaterials, ranging from basic science to host responses, as well as real-time applications. Some of the topics include but are not limited to: functional materials, smart materials, biomimetic materials, polymers, composites, ceramics, metals, alloys, and nanomaterials. This series will provide the most recent advances in biomedical materials, including design, synthesis, processing, and characterization. This series will accept both authored and edited volumes, including monographs, textbooks, reference works, and handbooks. This series aims to publish new advances in biomedical materials that have been made in the fabrication and development of biomaterials for different applications and the advancement of principles, theories, and designs. Each book title in the series will give a comprehensive overview of pioneering topics, and the readers will gain new knowledge and insights about the topic. As a collection, the series on 'Biomedical Materials for Multi-functional Applications' is anticipated to benefit a wide audience in academia, the research community, and industry.

Arnab Chanda · Dishant Sharma

Handbook of Artificial Tissues, Biofabrication and Bioprinting, Volume I

Springer

Arnab Chanda
Centre for Biomedical Engineering
Indian Institute of Technology (IIT) Delhi
New Delhi, Delhi, India

Dishant Sharma
Centre for Biomedical Engineering
Indian Institute of Technology (IIT) Delhi
New Delhi, Delhi, India

ISSN 2731-9695 ISSN 2731-9709 (electronic)
Biomedical Materials for Multi-functional Applications
ISBN 978-981-92-1306-1 ISBN 978-981-92-1307-8 (eBook)
https://doi.org/10.1007/978-981-92-1307-8

This Springer imprint is published by the registered company Springer Nature Singapore Pte Ltd.
The registered company address is: 152 Beach Road, #21-01/04 Gateway East, Singapore 189721, Singapore

Competing Interests The authors have no competing interests to declare that are relevant to the content of this manuscript.

Contents

Chapter 1
Artificial Tissues: History and Significance

1.1 Introduction

Artificial tissues, also known as engineered or synthetic tissues, are biological constructs designed to replicate the structure, function, and cellular environment of native human tissues. These constructs are typically fabricated using a combination of biomaterials, living cells, and biochemical cues through a process known as tissue engineering. The aim is to mimic the mechanical, structural, and physiological characteristics of natural tissues, thereby enabling their integration or functional replacement in biological systems [1, 2]. Artificial tissues may be entirely synthetic or semi-synthetic, often involving biodegradable scaffolds seeded with autologous, allogenic, or stem cells. Over time, these constructs can regenerate or support native tissue while gradually degrading or integrating into the body's natural architecture [3, 4]. Tissue engineering has evolved into a multidisciplinary field, combining principles from materials science, cell biology, biomedical engineering, and regenerative medicine. This convergence has enabled the development of increasingly complex tissue analogs that can serve as viable alternatives to damaged or diseased tissues. Importantly, artificial tissues are not limited to structural roles; they are often engineered to perform physiological and biochemical functions, such as secretion of hormones, contractility, or signal transduction, depending on the target tissue type [5–7].

1.1.1 Importance of Artificial Tissues in Medicine and Biotechnology

Artificial tissues represent a critical advancement in modern biomedicine and biotechnology, addressing several limitations of conventional medical treatments

A. Chanda and D. Sharma, *Handbook of Artificial Tissues, Biofabrication and Bioprinting, Volume I*, Biomedical Materials for Multi-functional Applications,
https://doi.org/10.1007/978-981-92-1307-8_1

such as donor organ shortages, immune rejection, and limited functionality of prosthetic devices. One of the most significant impacts is in regenerative medicine, where artificial tissues can be used to repair or replace damaged tissues, skin resulting from injury (see Fig. 1.1), degenerative diseases, or congenital disorders. Unlike mechanical implants, these tissue constructs are biologically active and can promote natural healing and regeneration processes [8]. In addition to therapeutic use, artificial tissues offer transformative potential in biopharmaceutical development and toxicology testing. Traditional preclinical drug testing relies heavily on animal models, which often fail to accurately predict human responses due to interspecies variability. Engineered tissue models, particularly those based on human cells, offer more physiologically relevant systems for evaluating drug efficacy and toxicity, thus reducing the need for animal testing and improving clinical translation. Furthermore, artificial tissues play a vital role in personalized medicine, where patient-derived cells can be used to create individualized tissue models for screening treatments or studying disease progression. This approach enhances the precision of medical interventions while minimizing adverse effects. From a biotechnological perspective, these tissues are integral to high-throughput screening platforms, microphysiological systems, and organ-on-a-chip technologies, all of which are central to the development of safer and more effective therapeutics [9, 10].

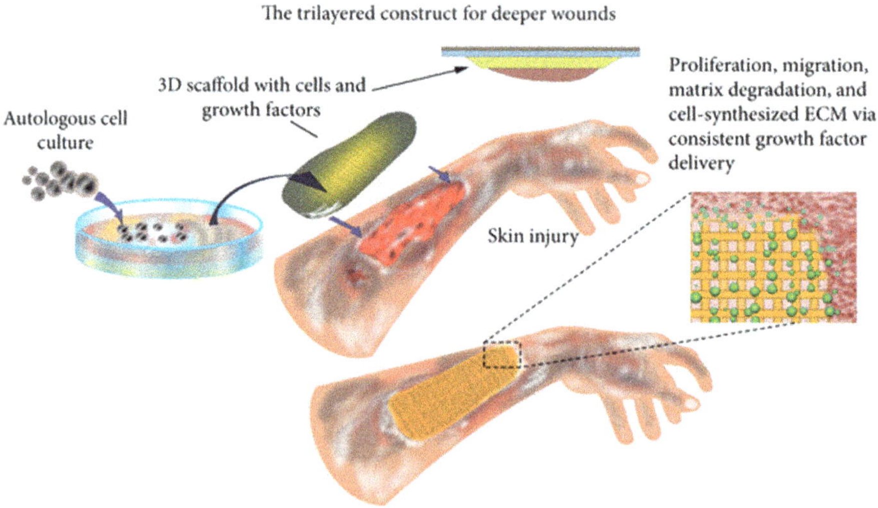

Fig. 1.1 Application of artificial tissue engineering in skin tissue engineering. Figure reproduced under license CC BY 4.0 [11]

1.1.2 Overview of Key Applications

Artificial tissues have found applications in a wide range of medical and research domains. Among the most prominent is tissue repair and regeneration, where constructs such as artificial skin, cartilage, bone, and blood vessels are used to restore function and structure in injured or degenerated tissues. For example, engineered skin substitutes are routinely used to treat burn patients, while artificial bone grafts aid in orthopedic reconstruction [12]. Another major application area is organ replacement. Although complete functional organs like the heart or liver are still in developmental stages, significant progress has been made in fabricating simpler organs such as the bladder and trachea. These bioengineered substitutes offer the promise of overcoming the limitations associated with donor organ availability and the risks of immune rejection [13]. In the field of drug testing and development, artificial tissues are used to create in vitro models that closely simulate human organ systems. Liver-on-a-chip and heart-on-a-chip systems, for instance, replicate metabolic and electrophysiological functions, respectively, and are employed in evaluating pharmacokinetics and cardiotoxicity. Such systems improve the predictive value of preclinical studies and help identify adverse effects earlier in the drug development pipeline [14]. Additionally, artificial tissues are increasingly employed in disease modeling, where they enable researchers to study the cellular and molecular mechanisms underlying various pathologies. These models are particularly valuable for conditions like cancer, neurodegenerative disorders, and rare genetic diseases, offering insights that are difficult to obtain from animal models or traditional 2D cultures [15–17].

1.2 Early Concepts of Artificial Tissues

The foundation of artificial tissue development is deeply rooted in early medical practices and material innovations that emerged long before modern tissue engineering. These preliminary efforts, particularly in skin grafting and organ substitutes, paved the way for contemporary artificial tissue systems.

1.2.1 Early Skin Grafting Techniques

One of the earliest documented forms of artificial tissue use is skin grafting, dating back to ancient civilizations. In 1500 BCE, Indian physician Sushruta described reconstructive surgical procedures involving autologous skin grafts for nose reconstruction following injury or amputation, often due to punitive measures [18]. In Europe, modern skin grafting began to formalize in the nineteenth century, particularly with Jacques-Louis Reverdin's successful use of small epidermal grafts in 1869, which he called "pinch grafts" [19, 20]. These developments laid the groundwork for understanding wound healing, tissue integration, and graft viability, concepts fundamental to modern tissue engineering.

1.2.2 The Beginnings of Artificial Organ Development

The mid-twentieth century saw early attempts to fabricate artificial organs to sustain life, especially for patients with end-stage organ failure. The invention of the artificial kidney (dialyzer) by Willem Kolff in the 1940s was a landmark innovation [21]. His rotating drum kidney, made from cellophane tubing and washing machine parts, allowed patients to survive acute renal failure for the first time. Similarly, early heart-lung machines developed by John Gibbon in the 1950s enabled open-heart surgeries and represented a convergence of physiology and mechanical engineering [22]. These milestones highlighted the importance of mimicking organ function, a principle that later extended into cellular and tissue-level constructs.

1.2.3 Development of Biocompatible Materials in the Twentieth Century

The evolution of artificial tissues was greatly influenced by the discovery and refinement of biocompatible materials. In the 1960s and 70s, polymers such as polytetrafluoroethylene (PTFE), polyurethane, and polylactic acid (PLA) emerged as key materials due to their non-toxicity, moldability, and degradation profiles [2]. These materials were essential in the fabrication of vascular grafts, bone cements, and wound dressings. Concurrently, silicone elastomers gained popularity for soft tissue implants, including breast and facial prostheses [23]. The integration of these materials into clinical practice emphasized the critical role of surface chemistry, mechanical compliance, and degradation behavior, cornerstones in modern scaffold design. Together, these early innovations reflect a trajectory from empirical interventions toward a rational, science-based engineering of tissues and organs. By the end of the twentieth century, interdisciplinary research had positioned artificial tissues as a viable frontier in regenerative medicine and biotechnology.

1.3 Evolution of Artificial Tissues in the Twentieth Century

The twentieth century marked a transformative era in the evolution of artificial tissues, driven by critical advancements in synthetic polymers, scaffold engineering, and cell and tissue culture techniques. Together, these breakthroughs formed the technological and scientific foundation of modern tissue engineering and regenerative medicine.

1.3.1 Development of Synthetic Polymers and Scaffolds

A cornerstone in the development of artificial tissues was the emergence of biocompatible synthetic polymers that could serve as scaffolds, three-dimensional structures designed to support cell adhesion, proliferation, and tissue formation. Early research focused on polymers such as polyglycolic acid (PGA) and polylactic acid (PLA) due to their biodegradability and minimal toxicity. These materials could be molded into porous structures capable of degrading into non-toxic byproducts while new tissue forms in their place [24]. The introduction of copolymers, particularly PLGA (a blend of PLA and PGA), enabled researchers to fine-tune the mechanical strength and degradation rate of scaffolds, thus improving their adaptability to different tissue types [25]. By the late 1980s, electrospinning and solvent casting techniques allowed for more precise fabrication of porous matrices that mimicked the extracellular matrix (ECM) in native tissues. These scaffolds not only provided mechanical support but also served as biochemical and topographical cues that guided cellular behavior [26–28]. The field saw another leap with the incorporation of hydrogels, such as polyethylene glycol (PEG) and alginate, which offered high water content and ECM-like viscoelasticity. Hydrogels supported encapsulated cell survival and enabled the controlled delivery of growth factors, enzymes, and drugs [29, 30]. These materials remain widely used today in cartilage repair, wound healing, and soft tissue engineering (Fig. 1.2).

1.3.2 Advances in Tissue Culture and Regenerative Medicine

Parallel to materials innovation was the revolution in tissue culture techniques, particularly the ability to isolate, expand, and differentiate various types of human cells in vitro. In 1952, Theodore Puck and Philip Marcus successfully cultured individual HeLa cells, laying the groundwork for clonal expansion and tissue formation from single-cell populations [32]. The 1960s and 70s witnessed the refinement of primary cell culture methods, allowing for the sustained growth of human fibroblasts, keratinocytes, and chondrocytes. A major milestone came in 1981 with the derivation of embryonic stem cells (ESCs) from mouse blastocysts by Martin Evans and

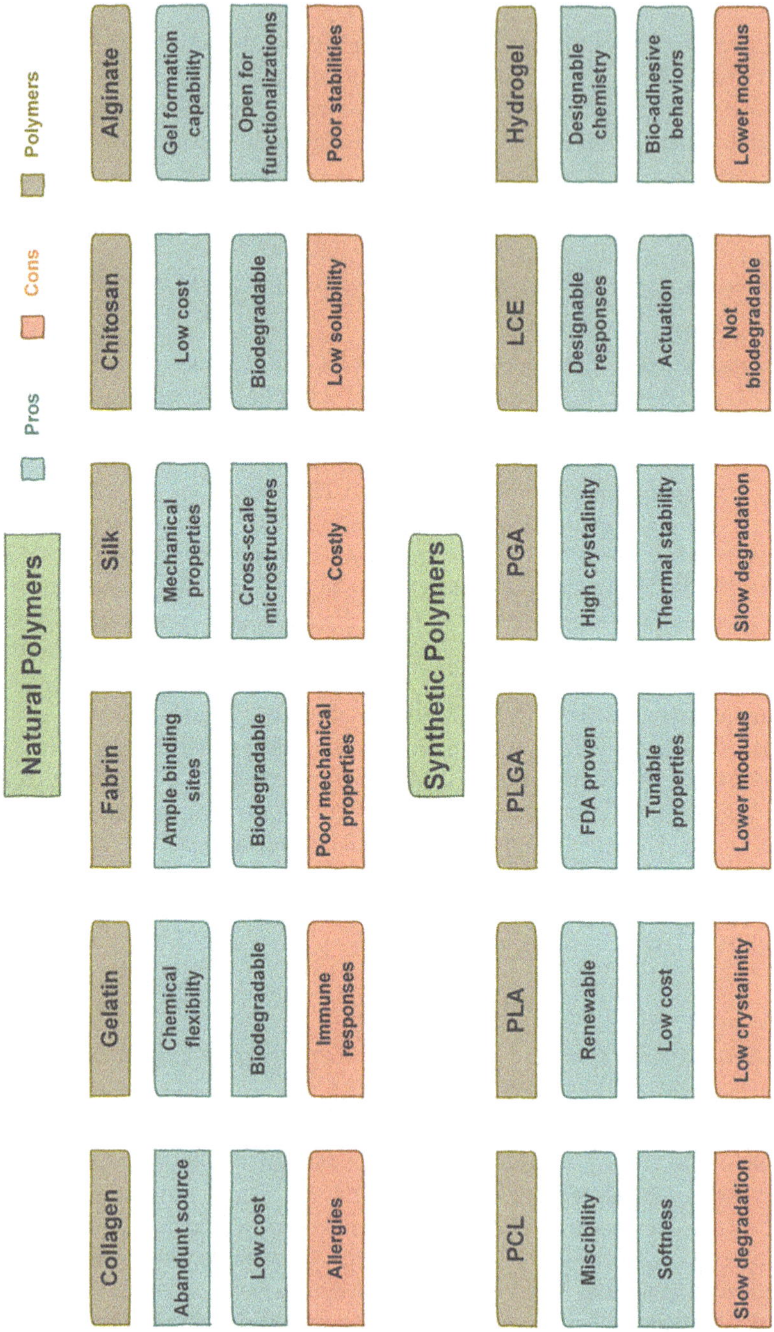

Fig. 1.2 Breakdown of natural and synthetic polymers utilized for tissue scaffolding. Figure reproduced under license CC BY 4.0 [31]

Matthew Kaufman, which introduced the concept of pluripotency into tissue engineering [33]. ESCs could differentiate into any cell type, offering unprecedented versatility in artificial tissue development. These advancements converged with the emergence of regenerative medicine, a field focused on restoring function to damaged tissues and organs through biological approaches. The 1990s saw the successful implantation of engineered skin, cartilage, and even urinary bladders into human patients [34–37]. In one landmark study, Atala et al. bioengineered bladders using autologous cells seeded on biodegradable scaffolds, which were then transplanted into pediatric patients with favorable long-term outcomes [38]. The growing understanding of cell signaling, ECM dynamics, and stem cell biology led to the development of more complex constructs, including co-cultures of multiple cell types and vascularized tissues. These artificial tissues not only provided mechanical functionality but also participated in immunomodulation, angiogenesis, and regeneration—essential features for clinical integration. By the end of the twentieth century, artificial tissues had evolved from rudimentary scaffolds to sophisticated, living systems capable of mimicking the form and function of native tissues. This evolution laid the groundwork for twenty-first-century advances in bioprinting, organ-on-a-chip technologies, and personalized tissue models.

1.4 Artificial Tissues in Regenerative Medicine

1.4.1 The Rise of Regenerative Medicine

Regenerative medicine emerged in the late twentieth century as a paradigm shift in healthcare, focusing not merely on replacing damaged tissues with artificial implants but on restoring or regenerating native tissue structure and function using biological approaches. The field integrates principles from stem cell biology, developmental biology, and tissue engineering to facilitate in vivo tissue regeneration or to develop functional tissue substitutes ex vivo. Coined in the early 1990s, the term "regenerative medicine" gained prominence with advancements in stem cell technologies, biomaterials, and cell delivery systems [39]. Unlike traditional artificial tissues, often limited to passive roles such as structural support, regenerative medicine leverages living cells, often seeded on scaffolds, to promote self-repair and functional integration within the host. Key to this transformation was the understanding that native tissue regeneration could be stimulated not just by implanting structural scaffolds, but by recreating the cellular microenvironment, including signaling molecules and extracellular matrix (ECM) components, that guide tissue morphogenesis and repair [40–43].

1.4.2 Regenerative Medicine Versus Traditional Artificial Tissues

Traditional artificial tissues, such as synthetic vascular grafts, orthopedic implants, or silicone-based prosthetics, often serve mechanical or cosmetic functions. These constructs, while biocompatible, typically do not promote intrinsic regeneration or cellular integration. They are subject to long-term complications such as immune rejection, infection, or mechanical failure. In contrast, regenerative tissue constructs aim to be bioactive and biomimetic, promoting angiogenesis, cell differentiation, and tissue remodeling. For example, regenerative scaffolds may incorporate growth factors, such as VEGF or BMP-2, to recruit endogenous stem cells or endothelial cells, thereby enhancing tissue regeneration in situ [44]. Moreover, regenerative tissues are increasingly designed to be patient-specific through autologous cell harvesting or induced pluripotent stem cell (iPSC) technology, reducing immunogenicity and enhancing long-term viability [45–47]. This distinction highlights a key shift: from replacement to regeneration, from passive to interactive, and from off-the-shelf to personalized solutions.

1.4.3 Clinical Breakthroughs and Applications

Several clinical breakthroughs in regenerative medicine illustrate the transformative potential of artificial tissues. One notable example is the successful implantation of tissue-engineered bladders into pediatric patients suffering from spina bifida. These constructs, made from autologous urothelial and muscle cells seeded onto biodegradable scaffolds, restored bladder function without triggering immune rejection. In another milestone, bioengineered tracheas were implanted into patients using a decellularized donor matrix reseeded with the patient's stem cells. These constructs maintained airway patency and epithelial lining, demonstrating feasibility for complex hollow organs. Similarly, engineered skin substitutes, such as Apligraf® and Dermagraft®, which combine fibroblasts, keratinocytes, and ECM components, have been approved for chronic wound healing and diabetic ulcers [48]. Regenerative approaches are also being explored in cardiac repair, where stem cell-laden patches or injectable hydrogels have been tested for myocardial infarction recovery. Early-phase trials have shown modest improvements in ventricular function and reduced scarring [49]. Despite these successes, challenges remain. Long-term durability, vascularization, and regulatory hurdles continue to limit widespread adoption. Nonetheless, the convergence of artificial tissue technologies with regenerative strategies promises a new era in medicine—one that aims not just to replace, but to heal [50–53].

1.5 Technological Breakthroughs in Artificial Tissue Development

The development of artificial tissues has rapidly accelerated in recent decades due to transformative innovations in 3D bioprinting and biomaterials science. These technologies aim to overcome the limitations of traditional scaffolding techniques and usher in a new era of complex, functional tissue constructs capable of clinical translation.

1.5.1 3D Bioprinting and Its Impact

3D bioprinting has emerged as a groundbreaking technology for fabricating artificial tissues with precise spatial architecture (see Fig. 1.3). Unlike conventional scaffold fabrication, bioprinting allows for the layer-by-layer deposition of living cells, biomaterials, and growth factors to create biomimetic structures that resemble native tissues. At the core of bioprinting are bioinks, formulations typically composed of hydrogels, cells, and bioactive molecules. Bioinks must possess properties such as biocompatibility, tunable mechanical strength, and printability. Common bioinks include alginate, gelatin-methacryloyl (GelMA), and collagen-based matrices, which provide a hydrated environment for encapsulated cells and support cellular activities such as adhesion and differentiation [54].

In recent years, researchers have succeeded in printing vascularized tissue constructs, such as perfusable liver lobules and cardiac patches, which mimic organ microarchitecture and allow for nutrient and oxygen transport [55–59]. Additionally, bioprinted skin substitutes and cartilage have entered preclinical and early clinical trials, demonstrating promising integration and healing outcomes. Despite these achievements, the field faces several challenges. The resolution and fidelity of bioprinted tissues remain limited, especially when replicating microvascular networks and neural interfaces. Furthermore, cell viability during printing, bioink standardization, and scalability for large tissues or organs present ongoing technical barriers. Nevertheless, advancements in multi-material printers, computational modeling, and stimuli-responsive bioinks are rapidly expanding the potential of bioprinting for regenerative medicine and personalized therapies.

1.5.2 Advances in Biomaterials

Parallel to bioprinting, significant progress in biomaterials engineering has expanded the toolkit for designing functional artificial tissues. Earlier materials, such as

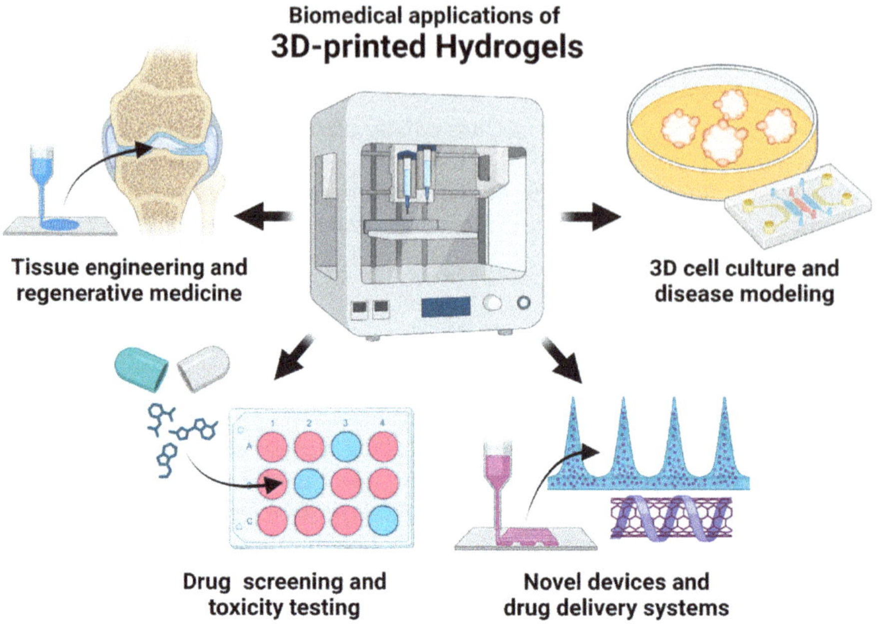

Fig. 1.3 A schematic representation of 3D bioprinting and its applications in biological domains. Reproduced under license CC by 4.0 [60] (https://creativecommons.org/licenses/by/4.0/)

PLA and PLGA, while biodegradable, were primarily passive and lacked biological signaling capability. Modern approaches emphasize the use of bioactive materials that can interact with host tissues and direct cellular responses. These include calcium phosphate ceramics for bone regeneration, decellularized extracellular matrix (dECM) materials that retain native growth factors and structural proteins, and smart hydrogels capable of responding to physiological stimuli (e.g., pH, temperature, enzymes) [61]. Such materials promote cell migration, angiogenesis, and immunomodulation, enhancing integration with the host and functional tissue regeneration. Recent innovations also include nanocomposite materials that integrate nanoparticles with polymers to enhance mechanical strength, conductivity, or antimicrobial properties. For example, incorporating graphene oxide or silicon nanowires into scaffolds can support nerve regeneration or cardiac tissue engineering by facilitating electrical signal conduction. Furthermore, the advent of biomimetic surface modifications, such as RGD peptide grafting or micro/nanopatterning, allows for tailored cell-material interactions. These surface cues are essential for guiding cell alignment, elongation, and tissue-specific function, especially in applications like tendon, muscle, and vascular tissue engineering [62–65]. As the field progresses, the synergy between 3D bioprinting and advanced biomaterials is expected to yield increasingly complex, vascularized, and innervated tissue constructs. The ability to integrate mechanical, chemical, and biological functionalities into artificial tissues is pivotal for their clinical translation and long-term performance.

1.6 Ethical and Societal Considerations

The development and application of artificial tissues, especially those integrated with living cells or derived from human biological materials, pose a variety of ethical, regulatory, and societal questions. As these technologies progress from laboratory research to clinical therapies, stakeholders must address concerns surrounding safety, consent, access, and public trust.

1.6.1 Ethical Questions About Artificial Tissues

Artificial tissues, particularly those involving stem cells, genetic engineering, or patient-derived biomaterials, raise fundamental ethical dilemmas. One key issue is the source of cells. While adult stem cells and induced pluripotent stem cells (iPSCs) present fewer ethical concerns, embryonic stem cells (ESCs) have long been controversial due to their derivation from human embryos, sparking debates over the moral status of early-stage human life [66]. Another major concern relates to informed consent for the use of human tissues. Donors must be clearly informed about how their biological samples will be used, especially if tissues are modified or commercialized. The potential for ownership disputes also arises, particularly when tissues lead to profitable therapies or patents. Moreover, the boundary between therapy and enhancement becomes blurred. Artificial tissues could potentially be engineered for non-therapeutic applications, such as increasing strength, endurance, or intelligence, raising questions about fairness, identity, and bioethics [67]. The possibility of creating entire organs or complex composite tissues, such as neural constructs or reproductive systems, also brings up philosophical and legal challenges concerning personhood, autonomy, and the extent to which the human body can or should be engineered.

1.6.2 Regulatory Challenges

The regulation of artificial tissues is complex due to their hybrid nature; they may be classified as medical devices, biologics, or combination products, depending on composition and intended use. This ambiguity complicates approval pathways and oversight. For instance, in the U.S., the Food and Drug Administration (FDA) uses multiple regulatory frameworks. Tissue-based products may be regulated under the Public Health Service Act (Section 361) or Section 351 if they are more than minimally manipulated or used for non-homologous functions [68]. Such classifications affect whether the product requires premarket approval, clinical trials, or post-market surveillance. In the European Union, products are often governed by Regulation (EC) No. 1394/2007 for Advanced Therapy Medicinal Products (ATMPs), which includes tissue-engineered products (TEPs) [69]. However, discrepancies in regulatory interpretation between regions can hinder global clinical translation and harmonization. Additionally, regulators face the challenge of balancing innovation with safety. Artificial tissues must be rigorously tested for biocompatibility, tumorigenicity, immunogenicity, and long-term performance. Yet overly stringent regulation can stifle innovation and delay patient access to life-saving treatments.

1.6.3 Societal Impact and Public Perception

The societal response to artificial tissue technologies is shaped by a mix of hope, skepticism, and ethical concern. On one hand, the public is generally supportive of regenerative medicine's potential to treat previously incurable diseases. Surveys have shown widespread optimism about the promise of stem cell-based therapies and bioengineered organs. However, public acceptance is contingent on transparency, equitable access, and ethical oversight. There is concern that such technologies may be available only to the wealthy, deepening healthcare inequalities. Ensuring universal access and insurance coverage for artificial tissue therapies will be key to their societal integration. Misinformation and unrealistic media portrayals—such as exaggerated timelines or "miracle cure" narratives—can distort public understanding and lead to disappointment or mistrust when clinical outcomes fall short [70]. Educating the public and fostering informed discourse are essential for building trust and engagement. Furthermore, there are cultural and religious perspectives that influence societal acceptance. For example, some religious groups may oppose the use of human-derived cells or synthetic body parts, viewing them as interfering with natural or divine order [71]. As artificial tissues become more prevalent in medicine and biotechnology, continuous engagement with bioethicists, regulators, patients, and the broader public is critical. The goal should not only be scientific progress, but socially responsible innovation.

1.7 Future Directions in Artificial Tissue Development

As artificial tissue engineering continues to evolve, future progress will hinge on the ability to overcome persistent technical limitations while simultaneously addressing emerging ethical challenges. The convergence of biofabrication technologies, advanced biomaterials, and cellular biology promises to unlock more clinically viable and personalized tissue substitutes. However, to realize this vision, multidisciplinary collaboration and regulatory foresight are essential.

1.7.1 Overcoming Technical Barriers

Despite significant strides in artificial tissue development, several key technical obstacles remain. One of the most pressing challenges is the vascularization of engineered tissues. Large tissue constructs require efficient oxygen and nutrient delivery, which in native organs is achieved through dense and hierarchical vasculature. Current efforts aim to integrate microvascular networks using advanced bioprinting, microfluidics, and angiogenic growth factor gradients [72–75]. Another major technical hurdle is achieving functional integration of artificial tissues with host systems. This includes innervation, mechanical synchronization (as in cardiac patches), and immune acceptance. Immunogenic responses, even with autologous or decellularized tissues, remain problematic. Solutions may involve immunomodulatory biomaterials, gene editing, or tolerance-inducing protocols [76]. Additionally, the fabrication of complex, multi-tissue interfaces, such as osteochondral units or skin-nerve-vascular composites, requires precise spatial organization and multi-cell type co-cultures. Novel biofabrication approaches, like 4D bioprinting, which allows printed tissues to change shape or function over time in response to stimuli, show promise in replicating such complex architectures. Standardization and scalability also pose significant barriers to clinical translation. There is a lack of standardized bioink formulations, scaffold properties, and quality control metrics across labs and manufacturers. Scalable production methods that maintain reproducibility and regulatory compliance will be essential for bringing engineered tissues from bench to bedside. The future will also see increased use of artificial intelligence (AI) and machine learning for predictive modeling of tissue behavior, optimizing scaffold design, and automating quality control in tissue manufacturing [77–80].

1.7.2 Ethical Considerations in Future Developments

As artificial tissues become increasingly sophisticated, ethical concerns will also evolve. The potential for whole organ engineering, especially brain or reproductive tissues, may blur the lines between repair, replacement, and enhancement, reigniting philosophical debates around identity and personhood [81]. One emerging issue is the development of organoids with neural activity. As brain organoids exhibit increasing complexity, questions arise about the moral status of such constructs, especially if they exhibit sentience-like behavior or pain perception. Ethical frameworks and oversight mechanisms will need to be established preemptively [82]. The integration of gene-editing tools, such as CRISPR-Cas9, into tissue engineering also raises concerns about germline modifications, especially in reproductive tissues or gametes. While somatic therapies are generally accepted, heritable changes could have unpredictable, long-term consequences and ethical implications [83]. Equity of access remains a future concern. Advanced therapies developed in high-income countries may remain inaccessible to those in low- and middle-income regions, widening global health disparities. Future policies must prioritize affordability, accessibility, and international collaboration to ensure that the benefits of artificial tissue technologies are distributed fairly [84]. Lastly, data privacy and biobanking of patient-derived cells or tissues pose new risks in an age of digitized healthcare. Robust informed consent, ownership rights, and data protection policies must accompany the storage and use of biological materials in tissue engineering.

1.8 Conclusions

The field of artificial tissue engineering has undergone transformative evolution, advancing from primitive grafting methods to the development of complex, functional biomimetic structures. Early experiments, such as autologous skin grafts and the first biocompatible materials, set the stage for the emergence of synthetic polymers and scaffold technologies in the twentieth century. These materials, coupled with breakthroughs in cell culture and regenerative biology, laid the groundwork for today's multifaceted tissue engineering approaches. In the twenty-first century, artificial tissues are no longer mere structural fillers but dynamic systems capable of biological integration and therapeutic function. Modern innovations such as 3D bioprinting, bioactive scaffolds, and organoids have expanded the potential applications of artificial tissues, from localized repair to whole organ regeneration and drug testing platforms [85, 86]. These developments have been paralleled by growing integration with regenerative medicine, where the boundary between repair and regeneration is increasingly blurred. At the same time, the field is experiencing a paradigm shift driven by technological, ethical, and regulatory considerations. Complex questions regarding safety, identity, accessibility, and societal perception must be addressed alongside the technical advances.

1.8.1 Significance of Artificial Tissues for Future Medical Advancements

Artificial tissues hold immense promise for revolutionizing healthcare across a broad spectrum of clinical challenges. Tissue shortages for transplantation, chronic degenerative diseases, and personalized medicine are among the areas where artificial tissues could offer transformative solutions. For instance, engineered cardiac patches and vascular grafts show potential to reduce the dependency on donor organs and lower transplant rejection rates. In drug discovery and toxicology, organ-on-a-chip and bioprinted tissue models can recapitulate human-specific responses, reducing the reliance on animal models and increasing the predictive value of preclinical testing [87] (see Fig. 1.4). Furthermore, artificial tissues are crucial for precision medicine, enabling therapies that are tailored to an individual's cellular and genetic makeup.

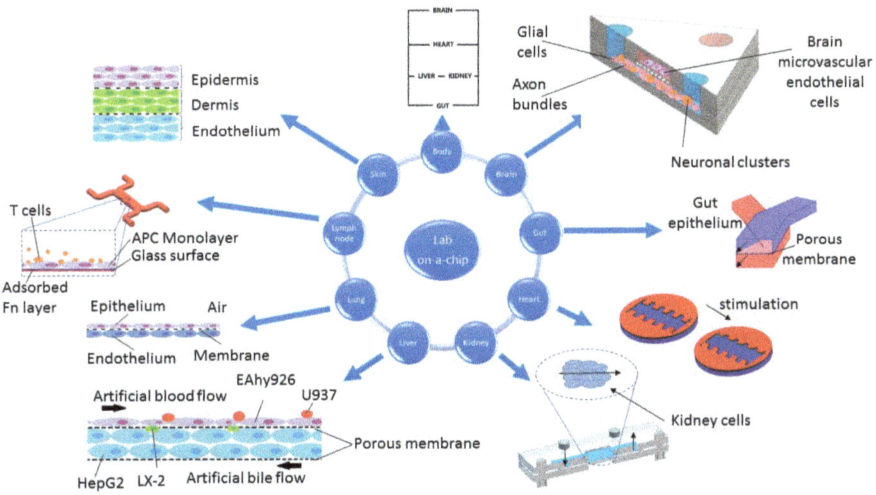

Fig. 1.4 Examples of lab-on-a-chip system applications include models replicating various human organs such as the body, brain, gut, heart, kidney, liver, lung, lymph node, and skin. Figure reproduced under license CC BY 4.0 [88]

The integration of artificial intelligence (AI) and data-driven modeling is expected to further enhance tissue engineering by enabling predictive design, optimizing scaffold properties, and simulating tissue behavior under physiological conditions.

1.8.2 The Road Ahead: New Frontiers in Artificial Tissues

Looking forward, several new frontiers in artificial tissue development are emerging. One of the most promising areas is whole-organ engineering, where the goal is not just to mimic tissue function but to recreate fully functional organs suitable for transplantation. The decellularization-recellularization approach and advances in perfusion bioreactors are bringing this goal closer to reality. Another frontier involves neurotissues and brain organoids, which are enabling new insights into neurological diseases and potential therapeutic interventions. However, this progress must be tempered with ethical vigilance, especially as constructs approach functional complexity that mimics cognition or sensation. Additionally, 4D bioprinting, wherein printed tissues respond dynamically to environmental stimuli, opens avenues for creating adaptive implants and smart scaffolds that evolve post-implantation. The future may also see hybrid bioelectronic tissues, merging biological constructs with electronic interfaces to enable real-time monitoring and control. Nevertheless, for these innovations to translate successfully into clinical use, regulatory harmonization, standardization, and global ethical frameworks will be essential. Challenges related to equity, consent, and long-term safety must be proactively addressed to ensure responsible and inclusive advancement of artificial tissue technologies [82]. In conclusion, artificial tissues represent one of the most exciting and impactful domains in modern medicine and biotechnology. Their continued development will not only redefine our therapeutic toolkit but also reshape our understanding of the human body and its potential for self-repair and augmentation.

References

1. Tezcaner A, Köse G, Hasirci V (2002) Fundamentals of tissue engineering: tissues and applications. Technol Health Care 10:203–216
2. Fisher JP, Mikos AG, Bronzino JD (1993) Tissue engineering. Science 260(5110):1–583. https://doi.org/10.1126/SCIENCE.8493529g
3. Hosseinkhani M et al (2014) Tissue engineered scaffolds in regenerative medicine. World J Plast Surg 3:3
4. Chanda A, Gupta S (2025) Healthcare entrepreneurship and management. Routledge, Taylor & Francis Group
5. Butler DL, Goldstein SA, Guilak F (2000) Functional tissue engineering: the role of biomechanics. J Biomech Eng 122:570–575
6. Gupta S, Singh G, Chanda A (2021) Prediction of diabetic foot ulcer progression: a computational study. Biomed Phys Eng Express 7:065020
7. Gupta S, Gupta V, Chanda A (2022) Biomechanical modeling of novel high expansion auxetic skin grafts. Int J Numer Method Biomed Eng 38:e3586
8. Lu L et al (2015) Tissue engineered constructs: perspectives on clinical translation. Ann Biomed Eng 43:796
9. Afazal M, Gupta S, Tevatia A, Afreen S, Chanda A (2023) Computational fluid dynamics-based model for assessing rupture risk in cerebral arteries with varying aneurysm sizes. Computation 11:79
10. Ellahi A, Gupta S, Bose D, Chanda A (2025) A high-fidelity biomechanical modeling framework for injury prediction during frontal car crash. Comput Methods Biomech Biomed Eng 28:13–24
11. Kaur A, Midha S, Giri S, Mohanty S (2019) Functional skin grafts: where biomaterials meet stem cells. Stem Cells Int 2019:1
12. Tompkins RG, Burke JF (1990) Progress in burn treatment and the use of artificial skin. World J Surg 14:819–824
13. Welman T, Michel S, Segaren N, Shanmugarajah K (2015) Bioengineering for organ transplantation: progress and challenges. Bioengineered 6:257–261
14. Tadevosyan K (2024) Heart-on-a-chip as biomimetic platform for cardiac physiology and drug toxicity testing. Tesis Dr. Facultat de Medicina i Ciències de la Salut
15. Benam KH et al (2015) Engineered in vitro disease models. Annu Rev Pathol Mech Dis 10:195–262
16. Singh G, Yadav P, Chanda A (2024) Development of biofidelic skin simulants based on fresh cadaveric skin tests. Eur Burn J 5:454–463
17. Yadav P, Kamboj M, Das B (2024) Application of nanotechnology in antimicrobial coating on surgical instruments. Appl Nanotechnol Biomed Eng 150–168. https://doi.org/10.1201/978 1003432661-9
18. Champaneria MC, Workman AD, Gupta SC (2014) Sushruta: father of plastic surgery. Ann Plast Surg 73:2–7
19. Kohlhauser M, Luze H, Nischwitz SP, Kamolz LP (2021) Historical evolution of skin grafting—a journey through time. Medicina (B Aires) 57:348

20. Yadav P et al (2025) Gelatin multiwalled carbon nanotube composite 3D printed semi biological mesh for abdominal hernia treatment. Chem Asian J 20:e202401136
21. Kolff WJ (1957) The artificial kidney; past, present, and future. Circulation 15:285–294
22. Gibbon JHJ (1954) Application of a mechanical heart and lung apparatus to cardiac surgery. Minn Med 37:171–185
23. Che Lah NF, Ahmad AL, Low SC, Shoparwe NF (2019) The role of porogen-polymer complexation in atrazine imprinted polymer to work as an electrochemical sensor in water. J Environ Chem Eng 7:103500
24. Cranin AN (1985) Biomaterials: an interfacial approach, L. L. Hench and E. C. Ethridge, New York, Academic, 1982, 384 pp. 14 Chapters, Glossary, Bibliography, and Index. Price: $42.00. J Biomed Mater Res 19:611–612
25. Pitt GG, Gratzl MM, Kimmel GL, Surles J, Sohindler A (1981) Aliphatic polyesters II. The degradation of poly (DL-lactide), poly (ε-caprolactone), and their copolymers in vivo. Biomaterials 2:215–220
26. Hutmacher DW (2000) Scaffolds in tissue engineering bone and cartilage. Biomaterials 21:2529–2543
27. Verma S, Singh G, Chanda A (2024) Development of a computational framework for determination of detrimental vibrations on the human spine segments. Multiscale Sci Eng 6(1):48–56
28. Verma S, Singh G, Chanda A (2023) A novel finite element model for the study of harmful vibrations on the aging spine. Computation 11:93
29. Kopeček J (2007) Hydrogel biomaterials: a smart future? Biomaterials 28:5185
30. Verma S, Chanda A (2024) State-of-the-art of finite element modelling of the human spine to study the impact of vibrations: a review. Int J Comput Methods Eng Sci Mech 25:225–247
31. Cao S, Bo R, Zhang Y (2023) Polymeric scaffolds for regeneration of central/peripheral nerves and soft connective tissues. Adv NanoBiomed Res 3
32. Puck TT, Marcus PI (1956) Action of X-rays on mammalian cells. J Exp Med 103:653–666
33. Evans MJ, Kaufman MH (1981) Establishment in culture of pluripotential cells from mouse embryos. Nature 292:154–156
34. Ashammakhi N et al (2022) Highlights on advancing frontiers in tissue engineering. Tissue Eng Part B Rev 28:633
35. Singh G, Chanda A (2024) Finite element modeling of diabetic foot: a state-of-the-art review. Eng Res Express 6:012507
36. Singh G, Gupta V, Chanda A (2022) Mechanical characterization of rotating triangle shaped auxetic skin graft simulants. Fac Univ Ser Mech Eng
37. Gupta V, Singh G, Chanda A (2023) Modeling of metamaterial based incision patterns for generating high expansions in skin grafts. Clin Biomech 110:106118
38. Atala A, Bauer SB, Soker S, Yoo JJ, Retik AB (2006) Tissue-engineered autologous bladders for patients needing cystoplasty. Lancet 367:1241–1246
39. Atala A (2012) Regenerative medicine strategies. J Pediatr Surg 47:17–28
40. Griffith LG, Naughton G (2002) Tissue engineering—current challenges and expanding opportunities. Science 295:1009
41. Jiang C et al (2022) Biomechanics of skin grafts: effect of pattern size, spacing and orientation. Eng Res Express 4:015006
42. Singh G, Chanda A (2024) Development and biomechanical testing of artificial surrogates for vaginal tissue. Adv Mater Process Technol. https://doi.org/10.1080/2374068X.2023.2198837
43. Chanda A, Gupta V, Gupta S (2024) Development and mechanical testing of auxetic incisions on human cadaveric skin, pp 89–99. https://doi.org/10.1007/978-981-97-4383-4_7
44. Langer RS, Vacanti JP (1999) Tissue engineering: the challenges ahead. Sci Am 280:86–89
45. Yamanaka S (2012) Induced pluripotent stem cells: past, present, and future. Cell Stem Cell 10:678–684
46. Gupta V, Chanda A (2023) Biomechanical modelling of hierarchical metamaterials for skin grafting. In: Materials horizons: from nature to nanomaterials (part F1471), pp 71–83

47. Gupta V, Chanda A (2021) Expansion potential of skin grafts with novel I-shaped auxetic incisions. Biomed Phys Eng Express 8:015016
48. Veves A, Falanga V, Armstrong DG, Sabolinski ML (2001) Graftskin, a human skin equivalent, is effective in the management of noninfected neuropathic diabetic foot ulcers: a prospective randomized multicenter clinical trial. Diabetes Care 24:290–295
49. Menasché P et al (2001) Myoblast transplantation for heart failure. Lancet 357:279–280
50. Gupta V, Gupta S, Chanda A (2023) Development of an ultra-low-cost planar biaxial tester for soft tissue characterization. Biomed Phys Eng Express 9:025011
51. Chhikara K, Gupta S, Bose D, Kataria C, Chanda A (2023) Development and trial of a multipurpose customized orthosis for activities of daily living in patients with spinal cord injury. Prosthesis 5:467–479
52. Gupta V, Singh G, Chanda A (2023) Development of hierarchical auxetic skin graft simulants with high expansion potential. Biomed Eng Adv 5:100087
53. Gupta V, Chanda A (2024) Mechanical characterization of alternating slit, I-shaped and rotating triangle based auxetic skin graft phantoms. Mech Adv Mater Struct. https://doi.org/10.1080/15376494.2023.2250782
54. Skardal A et al (2012) Bioprinted amniotic fluid-derived stem cells accelerate healing of large skin wounds. Stem Cells Transl Med 1:792–802
55. Hinton TJ et al (2015) Three-dimensional printing of complex biological structures by freeform reversible embedding of suspended hydrogels. Sci Adv 1:e1500758
56. Gupta V, Singh G, Gupta S, Chanda A (2023) Expansion potential of auxetic prosthetic skin grafts: a review. Eng Res Express 5:022003
57. Singh G, Gupta V, Chanda A (2022) Artificial skin with varying biomechanical properties. Mater Today Proc 62:3162–3166
58. Singh G, Chanda A (2024) Biofidelic gallbladder tissue surrogates. Adv Mater Process Technol. https://doi.org/10.1080/2374068X.2023.2198835
59. Afazal M, Afreen S, Chanda A (2023) Computational modelling and analysis of hard tissue behavior around 0.5 mm and 0.85 mm platform switched abutment using 3D finite element analysis. Forces Mech 13:100243
60. Barcena AJR, Dhal K, Patel P, Ravi P, Kundu S, Tappa K (2023) Current biomedical applications of 3D-printed hydrogels. Gels 10(1):8
61. Pati F et al (2014) Printing three-dimensional tissue analogues with decellularized extracellular matrix bioink. Nat Commun 5:3935
62. Dvir T, Timko BP, Kohane DS, Langer R (2010) Nanotechnological strategies for engineering complex tissues. Nat Nanotechnol 6(1):13–22
63. Bose D, Gupta S, Chanda A (2025) Scalable direct manufacturing of a functional multipurpose wrist-hand orthosis using 3D printing. Ann 3D Print Med 17:100186
64. Chanda A, Unnikrishnan V, Flynn Z, Lackey K (2017) Experimental study on tissue phantoms to understand the effect of injury and suturing on human skin mechanical properties. Proc Inst Mech Eng Part H J Eng Med 231:80–91
65. Singh G, Chanda A (2022) Biomechanical modeling of progressive wound healing: a computational study. Biomed Eng Adv 4:100055
66. Lo B, Parham L (2009) Ethical issues in stem cell research. Endocr Rev 30:204
67. Michael J. The case against perfection: ethics in the age of genetic engineering. Sandel. https://sandel.scholars.harvard.edu/publications/case-against-perfection-ethics-age-genetic-engineering
68. FDA. Regulatory considerations for human cells, tissues, and cellular and tissue-based products: minimal manipulation and homologous use. https://www.fda.gov/regulatory-information/search-fda-guidance-documents/regulatory-considerations-human-cells-tissues-and-cellular-and-tissue-based-products-minimal
69. Regulation—1394/2007—EN—EUR-Lex. https://eur-lex.europa.eu/eli/reg/2007/1394/oj/eng
70. Petersen A, Anderson A, Allan S (2005) Science fiction/science fact: medical genetics in news stories. New Genet Soc 24:337–353

71. Campbell CS (1998) Religion and the body in medical research. Kennedy Inst Ethics J 8:275–305
72. Kong Z, Wang X (2023) Bioprinting technologies and bioinks for vascular model establishment. Int J Mol Sci 24:891
73. Chanda A (2018) Biomechanical modeling of human skin tissue surrogates. Biomimetics 3:18
74. Chanda A, Flynn Z, Unnikrishnan V (2018) Biomechanical characterization of normal and prolapsed vaginal tissue surrogates. J Mech Med Biol 18:1750100
75. Gupta V, Chanda A (2023) Auxetic incisions with alternating slit shapes: a promising technique for enhancing synthetic skin grafts expansion. Mater Res Express 10:075802
76. Wiles K, Fishman JM, De Coppi P, Birchall MA (2016) The host immune response to tissue-engineered organs: current problems and future directions. Tissue Eng Part B Rev 22:208–219
77. Bagherpour R, Bagherpour G, Mohammadi P (2024) Application of artificial intelligence in tissue engineering. Tissue Eng Part B Rev 31
78. Chanda A, Ruchti T, Unnikrishnan V (2018) Computational modeling of wound suture: a review. IEEE Rev Biomed Eng 11:165–176
79. Gupta V, Singla R, Chanda A (2023) Development and characterization of novel anisotropic skin graft simulants. Dermato 3:114–130
80. Chhikara K, Gupta S, Chanda A (2022) Development of a novel foot orthosis for plantar pain reduction. Mater Today Proc 62:3532–3537
81. Douglas T, Savulescu J (2010) Synthetic biology and the ethics of knowledge. J Med Ethics 36:687
82. Hyun I, Scharf-Deering JC, Lunshof JE (2020) Ethical issues related to brain organoid research. Brain Res 1732:146653
83. What are the ethical concerns of genome editing? https://www.genome.gov/about-genomics/policy-issues/Genome-Editing/ethical-concerns
84. Hermerén G (2021) The ethics of regenerative medicine. Biol Futur 72:113–118
85. Moroni L et al (2018) Biofabrication: a guide to technology and terminology. Trends Biotechnol 36:384–402
86. Malda J et al (2013) 25th anniversary article: engineering hydrogels for biofabrication. Adv Mater 25:5011–5028
87. Beyond animal testing: the rise of organs-on-chips technology. https://clarivate.com/life-sciences-healthcare/blog/beyond-animal-testing-the-rise-of-organs-on-chips-technology/
88. Klak M et al (2020) Novel strategies in artificial organ development: what is the future of medicine? Micromachines 11:646

Chapter 2
Anatomy of Tissues

2.1 Introduction

2.1.1 *Definition of Tissues*

Tissues are structured assemblies of similar or diverse cells that cooperate to perform specific physiological functions (see Fig. 2.1). These cellular aggregates are embedded within an extracellular matrix (ECM) that provides structural and biochemical support, enabling tissues to maintain homeostasis, facilitate repair, and adapt to environmental demands. In the human body, tissues represent the intermediate level of biological organization, between cells and organs, and are essential to systemic function and integrity. They are not merely passive structures but are dynamic, capable of self-renewal, regeneration, and remodeling under both normal and pathological conditions [1–3].

2.1.2 *Classification of Tissues Based on Function*

Tissues in the human body are broadly classified into four primary categories based on their function: epithelial, connective, muscle, and nervous tissues. Each category fulfills distinct physiological roles, which are crucial for understanding tissue behavior in both native and engineered systems. Epithelial tissue forms protective layers that cover body surfaces and line cavities and hollow organs. These tissues are tightly packed, avascular, and highly regenerative. They serve functions such as absorption, secretion, filtration, and protection. Epithelia can be simple (single-layered) or stratified (multi-layered), with specialized variants like columnar, cuboidal, and squamous types based on cellular morphology [5–7]. Connective tissue is the most diverse category, encompassing loose and dense connective tissues,

A. Chanda and D. Sharma, *Handbook of Artificial Tissues, Biofabrication and Bioprinting, Volume I*, Biomedical Materials for Multi-functional Applications,
https://doi.org/10.1007/978-981-92-1307-8_2

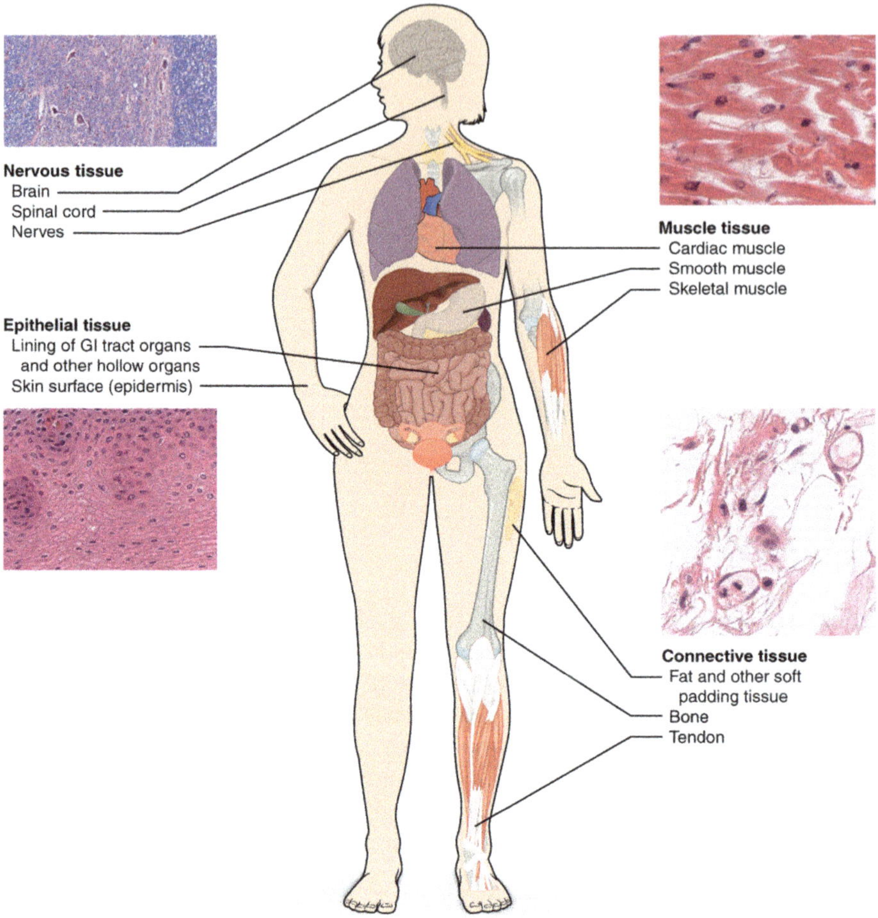

Fig. 2.1 A diagram illustrating the four main types of human tissue, nervous, epithelial, muscle, and connective, along with their locations and microscopic structures. Figure reproduced under CC BY-SA 4.0 [4] (https://creativecommons.org/licenses/by-sa/4.0/)

adipose tissue, cartilage, bone, and blood. Its primary function is to support and bind other tissues, while also playing roles in nutrient storage, immune defense, and tissue repair. The ECM composition, rich in collagen, elastin, and proteoglycans, confers tensile strength, elasticity, and resilience [8, 9]. Muscle tissue is specialized for contraction and includes skeletal, cardiac, and smooth muscle types. These tissues convert chemical energy into mechanical work, enabling voluntary movements (skeletal), involuntary rhythmic contractions (cardiac), and internal peristalsis (smooth). Muscle tissue is characterized by its high metabolic activity and responsiveness to electrical stimuli. Other soft tissues, such as nervous tissue, consist of neurons and glial cells. Nervous tissue facilitates rapid communication through electrical and chemical signaling and is integral to sensation, cognition, and motor control. Due to its complexity and limited regenerative capacity, nervous tissue presents unique challenges in both natural healing and artificial reconstruction.

2.1.3 *Importance of Tissue Anatomy in Artificial Tissue Engineering*

An in-depth understanding of tissue anatomy is fundamental to the development of artificial tissues in regenerative medicine and biomedical engineering. Tissue engineering aims to restore, maintain, or improve tissue function by integrating cells, biomaterials, and bioactive molecules. Anatomical knowledge guides scaffold design, cellular sourcing, and bioreactor conditioning by defining the spatial arrangement, mechanical properties, and microenvironmental cues necessary for functional tissue regeneration [10, 11]. For instance, replicating the layered architecture of epithelial tissues or the anisotropic organization of muscle fibers requires precise anatomical modeling. Additionally, insights into the vascularization and innervation patterns of native tissues are critical for fabricating viable large-scale constructs. Misunderstanding or oversimplifying tissue anatomy can result in poorly integrated implants, immune rejection, or limited physiological function. Moreover, advances in histology and imaging technologies have enabled high-resolution visualization of tissue architecture, fostering the development of anatomically faithful models. These models are instrumental in drug testing, disease modeling, and the replacement of damaged tissues, making anatomical fidelity not just a design criterion but a prerequisite for clinical translation [12–14]. A detailed comprehension of tissue anatomy forms the foundation of both biological understanding and tissue engineering innovation. The alignment of anatomical principles with engineering methodologies paves the way for more effective, biomimetic, and functional artificial tissues.

2.2 Overview of Natural Tissue Structure and Function

2.2.1 *Cellular and Extracellular Components*

Biological tissues are composed of two principal elements: cells and the extracellular matrix (ECM). These components are intimately linked in function and organization, working synergistically to maintain tissue integrity, facilitate communication, and support physiological roles. Understanding both cellular and ECM contributions is essential to replicating native tissue characteristics in artificial systems.

2.2.2 Cells and Their Roles in Tissue Function

Cells serve as the fundamental living units of tissues. Their primary roles vary depending on tissue type but generally include proliferation, signaling, matrix secretion, immune modulation, and mechanical support. In epithelial tissues, for instance, cells act as barriers and regulators of selective permeability, while in connective tissues, fibroblasts synthesize collagen and elastin, maintaining ECM homeostasis [15, 16]. In muscular tissues, myocytes facilitate contraction, and in nervous tissues, neurons transmit electrical impulses, enabling intercellular communication.

Furthermore, tissue-specific stem cells play a pivotal role in regeneration and repair. These cells, often residing in niches, can differentiate into specialized cells when prompted by injury or developmental signals. Cellular diversity, ranging from immune cells in connective tissues to specialized endothelial cells in vasculature, enhances the functional versatility of tissues [17–19].

2.2.3 Extracellular Matrix (ECM): Composition and Function

The ECM is a dynamic, three-dimensional network of macromolecules secreted by cells, providing not only mechanical scaffolding but also critical biochemical and biomechanical cues. It consists of structural proteins such as collagen and elastin, glycoproteins like fibronectin and laminin, and proteoglycans rich in glycosaminoglycans (GAGs) [20]. These components endow tissues with elasticity, tensile strength, and hydration.

The ECM governs key cellular behaviors such as adhesion, proliferation, migration, and differentiation via mechanotransduction and integrin signaling pathways. Its degradation and remodeling, regulated by matrix metalloproteinases (MMPs), are vital for tissue development, wound healing, and pathological processes such as cancer metastasis [21].

2.2.4 Tissue Hierarchy

Biological tissues exhibit a hierarchical organization that spans from microscopic to macroscopic levels. This hierarchical structure underlies the integrated functionality of organs and organ systems and is essential to recapitulate in engineered constructs for them to perform physiologically.

2.2.5 Cellular Level

At the cellular level, tissues are composed of individual cells with specific phenotypes, morphologies, and intracellular machinery. These cells are often polarized (e.g., epithelial cells), responsive to extracellular stimuli, and capable of interacting through junctional complexes and signaling molecules. Cellular arrangements, whether in clusters, layers, or dispersed within the ECM, affect overall tissue mechanics and behavior [22].

2.2.6 Tissue Level

The tissue level is characterized by the coordinated organization of multiple cell types and their ECM in spatial and functional harmony. For example, skeletal muscle tissue exhibits aligned fibers interspersed with satellite cells and capillaries, optimizing it for contraction and regeneration. The orientation, density, and matrix alignment at this level contribute significantly to a tissue's mechanical properties and physiological performance [23].

2.2.7 Organ and System Levels

At the organ level, various tissue types integrate to form complex structures capable of executing specific functions. The heart, for example, combines muscle tissue (myocardium), connective tissue, and endothelial lining to generate and regulate blood flow. Organs then work together in systems, such as the circulatory or respiratory systems, illustrating the culmination of tissue hierarchy into coordinated biological function [24–26]. Understanding this multiscale tissue hierarchy is critical for designing artificial tissues that emulate native function. Failure to replicate a hierarchical organization may result in constructs that are structurally unstable or functionally inadequate. The natural structure and function of tissues are products of intricate cellular and extracellular interactions, reinforced by a hierarchical architecture. A comprehensive understanding of these elements—from molecular signaling to system-level integration—is indispensable for advancing tissue engineering and regenerative medicine.

2.3 Connective Tissues

2.3.1 General Characteristics of Connective Tissues

Connective tissues are one of the four primary tissue types in the human body and are characterized by their ability to support, bind, and protect other tissues and organs. Unlike epithelial tissues, which are cellularly dense, connective tissues typically contain fewer cells and a substantial extracellular matrix (ECM). This matrix, composed of fibrous proteins like collagen and elastin, ground substance, and glycoproteins, provides structural integrity, elasticity, and biochemical signaling [20].

These tissues exhibit varying degrees of vascularization and cellularity depending on their type and function. Resident cells such as fibroblasts, adipocytes, chondrocytes, osteocytes, and hematopoietic cells perform key functions, including matrix synthesis, energy storage, immune defense, and mineral deposition [27, 28].

2.3.2 Types of Connective Tissues

Connective tissues are classified into several types based on the density and arrangement of their cellular and matrix components. These include loose connective tissue, dense connective tissue, cartilage, bone, and blood.

2.3.3 Loose Connective Tissue (e.g., Areolar, Adipose)

Loose connective tissue is characterized by a loosely arranged matrix with high water content and widely dispersed cells. Areolar tissue consists of fibroblasts embedded in a matrix of collagen and elastic fibers, providing cushioning and flexibility around organs, blood vessels, and nerves. Adipose tissue, dominated by lipid-storing adipocytes, plays roles in energy storage, insulation, and endocrine signaling. Figure 2.2 highlighting key components such as collagenous and elastic fibers, cell nuclei, chondrocytes within chondroitin sulfate, and blood cells in plasma, demonstrating their structural and functional roles in the human body.

2.3.4 Dense Connective Tissue (e.g., Tendons, Ligaments)

Dense connective tissue has a tightly packed collagen fiber matrix that imparts high tensile strength. Tendons, which connect muscles to bones, and ligaments, which link bones to each other, are both examples. Fibroblasts in these tissues align along

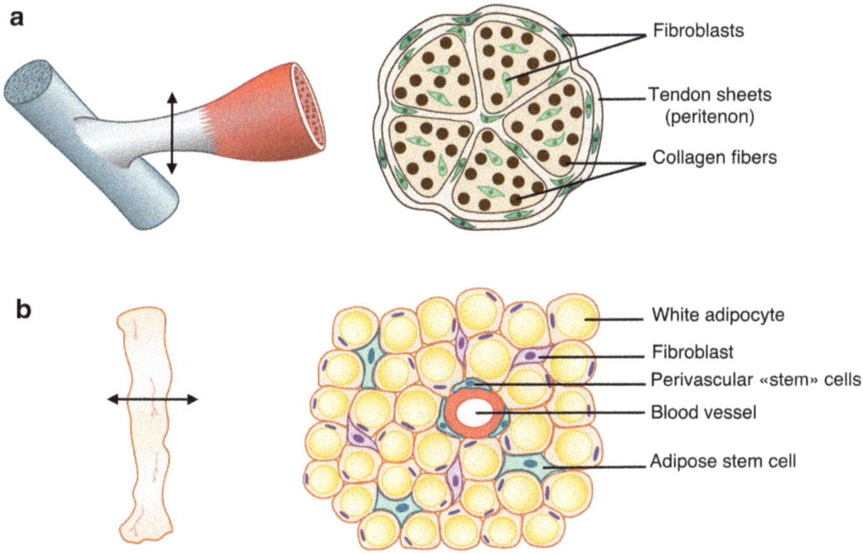

Fig. 2.2 Various types of connective tissue, including dense regular connective tissue, the tendon (**a**), and a loose connective tissue, the adipose tissue (**b**). Figure reproduced under license CC-BY-4.0 [29] (https://creativecommons.org/licenses/by/4.0/)

the direction of mechanical stress, producing organized collagen bundles suited to their mechanical role in transmitting force and maintaining joint stability [30–33].

2.3.5 Cartilage and Bone

Cartilage is a semi-rigid tissue composed of chondrocytes embedded in a dense ECM of type II collagen and proteoglycans. It is avascular, limiting its regenerative capacity, and provides flexible support in structures like the ear, nose, and joints. Bone tissue, in contrast, is highly mineralized with calcium phosphate crystals deposited around collagen fibers, making it rigid and supportive. Osteoblasts, osteoclasts, and osteocytes orchestrate bone remodeling and homeostasis [34].

2.3.6 Blood as a Specialized Connective Tissue

Blood is considered a specialized connective tissue due to its origin in the mesoderm and its function in transport and immunity. Its ECM is the plasma, which carries nutrients, hormones, and waste products. The cellular component includes erythrocytes for oxygen transport, leukocytes for immune defense, and platelets for clotting.

2.3.7 Artificial Connective Tissues

The engineering of artificial connective tissues has gained momentum due to the need for replacements in orthopedic, cardiovascular, and reconstructive medicine. These efforts aim to replicate the mechanical, biochemical, and functional properties of native tissues.

2.3.8 Artificial Cartilage, Bone, and Blood Substitutes

Artificial cartilage is being developed using hydrogels, electrospun fibers, and nanocomposites to mimic the viscoelastic and load-bearing properties of native cartilage. Scaffold materials such as polyethylene glycol (PEG), polylactic acid (PLA), and collagen are often used to support chondrocyte growth and matrix production. Bone tissue engineering typically involves biomimetic scaffolds composed of bioceramics like hydroxyapatite or β-tricalcium phosphate, which encourage osteogenic differentiation and mineral deposition. Incorporation of growth factors like bone morphogenetic proteins (BMPs) further enhances regeneration. Artificial blood substitutes, such as hemoglobin-based oxygen carriers (HBOCs) and perfluorocarbon emulsions, have been developed to address shortages in the blood supply and reduce immunogenicity. While challenges remain regarding toxicity and oxygen affinity, these substitutes have shown promise in trauma and surgical applications [35–38]. Connective tissues are integral to structural support, nutrient distribution, and tissue repair across all organ systems. A thorough understanding of their native properties has guided the development of artificial analogs, which continue to evolve through advances in biomaterials, stem cell technology, and tissue engineering. These innovations hold significant promise for regenerative medicine and translational therapies.

2.4 Muscle Tissues

2.4.1 Structure and Function of Muscle Tissues

Muscle tissues are specialized for contraction, enabling movement and force generation within the body. They are categorized into three distinct types: skeletal, cardiac, and smooth muscles, each with unique structural and functional characteristics.

Skeletal Muscle: These muscles are attached to bones and facilitate voluntary movements. They are composed of long, multinucleated fibers with a striated appearance due to the organized arrangement of actin and myosin filaments. Skeletal muscles are under conscious control and are essential for locomotion and posture maintenance [39].

Cardiac Muscle: Found exclusively in the heart, cardiac muscle fibers are striated like skeletal muscles but are branched and interconnected via intercalated discs. These discs contain gap junctions that allow for synchronized contractions, essential for effective heartbeats. Cardiac muscle operates involuntarily, with rhythmic contractions regulated by the heart's intrinsic pacemaker and autonomic nervous system [40].

Smooth Muscle: Located in the walls of hollow organs such as the intestines, blood vessels, and the bladder, smooth muscle fibers are spindle-shaped and lack striations. These muscles contract involuntarily, controlling movements like peristalsis in the digestive tract and vasoconstriction in blood vessels [41–44].

2.4.2 Cellular Organization of Muscle Tissues

At the cellular level, muscle tissues are composed of specialized cells called myocytes or muscle fibers. These fibers contain myofibrils, which are further organized into repeating units known as sarcomeres—the fundamental contractile units of muscle. Sarcomeres: Each sarcomere is delineated by Z-lines and comprises interlacing thick (myosin) and thin (actin) filaments. During contraction, the sliding filament theory explains that myosin heads bind to actin filaments, pulling them inward and shortening the sarcomere, leading to muscle contraction. This process is ATP-dependent and regulated by calcium ions, troponin, and tropomyosin complexes.

2.4.3 Types of Muscle Contraction

Muscle contractions can be classified based on their control mechanisms and the changes they produce in muscle length and tension.

Voluntary Contractions: These are consciously initiated movements, primarily involving skeletal muscles. Examples include walking, lifting objects, and speaking.

Involuntary Contractions: These occur without conscious control and involve both smooth and cardiac muscles. Functions such as heartbeat regulation, digestion, and blood vessel constriction are governed by involuntary contractions [45–47].

Further classification includes:

- Isometric Contractions: Muscle tension is generated without a change in muscle length, as seen when holding a heavy object stationary [48].

- Isotonic Contractions: Muscle changes length while maintaining constant tension. This includes:
  - Concentric Contractions: Muscle shortens while generating force, such as lifting a weight.
  - Eccentric Contractions: Muscle lengthens under tension, like lowering a weight slowly [48].

2.4.4 Artificial Muscle Tissues

Advancements in tissue engineering have led to the development of artificial muscle tissues, aiming to replicate the structure and function of natural muscles for medical and technological applications.

Bioactuators: These are engineered muscle constructs that respond to electrical or chemical stimuli, producing movement. They are utilized in soft robotics and prosthetics to mimic natural muscle actions.

Engineered Muscle Constructs: Researchers have developed methods to cultivate muscle tissues in vitro using scaffolds and bioreactors. These constructs can contract and generate force, offering potential treatments for muscle loss due to injury or disease. Recent innovations include 3D bioprinting techniques that allow for the precise arrangement of muscle cells and extracellular matrix components, enhancing the functionality of engineered muscles. Such constructs have demonstrated the ability to contract in multiple directions, closely resembling natural muscle behavior [49–52]. Muscle tissues are integral to numerous physiological processes, from voluntary movements to vital involuntary functions. Understanding their complex structure and contraction mechanisms has been pivotal in biomedical research. The emergence of artificial muscle tissues holds promise for regenerative medicine and the development of responsive prosthetics and robotics, bridging the gap between biological systems and engineered solutions.

2.5 Functional Soft Tissues

Functional soft tissues in the human body exhibit a wide spectrum of mechanical properties, particularly in terms of stiffness, which is crucial for their respective physiological roles. Stiffness, often quantified by Young's modulus, determines how a tissue deforms under mechanical stress. This chapter categorizes soft tissues based on their stiffness into low, medium, and high stiffness groups, providing insights into their structural characteristics and functional significance [53–56].

2.5.1 Tissues with Low Stiffness

Low-stiffness tissues are highly compliant and capable of significant deformation, which is essential for their protective and cushioning functions. These tissues typically have a Young's modulus ranging from a few hundred pascals to several kilopascals.

- **Brain Tissue**: The brain is among the softest tissues, with an elastic modulus of approximately 100 Pa. Its softness facilitates the absorption of mechanical shocks, protecting neural structures from injury [57].
- **Liver Tissue**: The liver exhibits slightly higher stiffness, with a modulus between 400 and 600 Pa. This compliance allows it to accommodate blood flow and metabolic processes efficiently [58].
- **Adipose Tissue**: Subcutaneous fat has a modulus ranging from 2 to 5 kPa, providing insulation and energy storage while cushioning underlying structures [59].

The low stiffness of these tissues is attributed to their high water content and minimal fibrous protein composition, enabling them to fulfill roles that require flexibility and shock absorption.

2.5.2 Tissues with Medium Stiffness

Medium-stiffness tissues balance flexibility and structural support, with Young's modulus values typically between 10 kPa and 1 MPa. This category includes:

- **Muscle Tissue**: Skeletal muscles have a modulus ranging from 10 to 100 kPa, allowing for contraction and force generation while maintaining compliance [60].
- **Skin**: Human skin exhibits a modulus between 0.42 and 0.85 MPa, providing a protective barrier while accommodating movement and environmental interactions [61].
- **Cartilage**: Articular cartilage, found in joints, has a modulus ranging from 0.5 to 0.9 MPa. Its viscoelastic properties enable it to withstand compressive forces during movement [62].

These tissues contain a higher proportion of structural proteins like collagen and elastin, contributing to their increased stiffness and functional versatility.

2.5.3 Tissues with High Stiffness

High-stiffness soft tissues are designed to resist substantial mechanical loads, with Young's modulus values exceeding 1 MPa. Key examples include:

- **Tendons**: Tendons exhibit a modulus ranging from 1.2 to 1.8 GPa, facilitating the transmission of muscular forces to bones [63].
- **Ligaments**: Ligaments have a modulus between 300 and 500 MPa, providing joint stability by connecting bones [64].

Although not a soft tissue, **bone** is often used as a reference, with a modulus of approximately 20 GPa, to mark the upper limit of biological stiffness.

The high stiffness of these tissues is due to their dense collagen fiber arrangement and, in the case of bone, mineralization, which confer the necessary mechanical strength for load-bearing functions. The mechanical properties of soft tissues are intricately linked to their biological functions. Understanding the stiffness characteristics of various tissues aids in the development of biomaterials, prosthetics, and tissue engineering strategies that aim to replicate or restore native tissue functions. Future research should continue to explore the complex interplay between tissue composition, structure, and mechanical behavior to advance medical science and engineering applications [65–67].

2.6 Comparative Anatomy of Natural and Artificial Tissues

2.6.1 Differences in Structural Properties Between Natural and Artificial Tissues

Natural tissues exhibit intricate hierarchical structures, spanning nanoscale to macroscale organization. This complexity facilitates specific mechanical properties, cellular interactions, and biological functions. For example, the extracellular matrix (ECM) in natural tissues provides structural support alongside biochemical cues essential for cell signaling and tissue homeostasis [68]. In contrast, artificial tissues, often engineered from synthetic polymers, attempt to replicate these properties but face challenges in mimicking the exact structural intricacies of natural tissues. Synthetic polymers offer tunable mechanical properties and controlled degradation rates but may lack the inherent bioactivity and cell recognition sites present in natural ECM components, affecting cell adhesion and proliferation [69]. Furthermore, natural tissues possess anisotropic mechanical properties tailored to their functions, a feature difficult to replicate in artificial constructs. The absence of native-like vascular networks in artificial tissues limits their ability to maintain cell viability and functionality over time [70]. For example, while natural cartilage or bone exhibit a complex collagen fiber orientation and mineralization gradient, artificial substitutes often display more homogeneous structures, which may impact their mechanical performance and integration.

2.6.2 Functional Considerations for Artificial Tissue Development

Developing artificial tissues requires understanding the functional needs of the target tissue. Key factors include mechanical strength, elasticity, biocompatibility, and support for cell adhesion and proliferation. Scaffold design is critical, as the scaffold must provide an appropriate structural framework that mimics the mechanical properties of native tissue while enabling biocompatibility and proper degradation rates [71]. The incorporation of bioactive molecules such as growth factors can enhance cellular responses and promote tissue integration. Bioreactors that provide mechanical stimulation and nutrient perfusion improve engineered tissue maturation and function [72–74]. Advances in 3D bioprinting have enabled the precise placement of cells and biomaterials to fabricate complex tissue structures. However, achieving the necessary resolution and fidelity to replicate native tissue architecture remains a significant challenge. This precision is essential for reproducing the cellular microenvironment and mechanical anisotropy characteristic of many natural tissues. Figure 2.3 represents the comparison of the mechanical properties of tissues versus biomaterials. The upper panel presents the Young's modulus values of different biological tissues, while the lower panel shows the corresponding values for commonly used biomaterials in tissue engineering.

2.6.3 Limitations in Artificial Tissues Relative to Natural Counterparts

Despite progress, artificial tissues often do not fully replicate the function of natural tissues. A major limitation is the lack of vascularization in engineered tissues, which restricts nutrient and oxygen delivery, leading to necrosis in tissue cores. Additionally, immune responses to implants can cause inflammation and fibrosis, impeding tissue integration and function. Though synthetic materials can be designed to minimize immune reactions, they may lack the immunomodulatory properties inherent to natural tissues [76]. Replicating the dynamic remodeling capacity of natural tissues also remains challenging. Natural tissues adapt to mechanical and biochemical cues through continuous remodeling, a feature artificial tissues currently cannot fully emulate. The long-term stability and function of artificial tissues remain concerns, as degradation byproducts and mechanical wear can compromise performance [77].

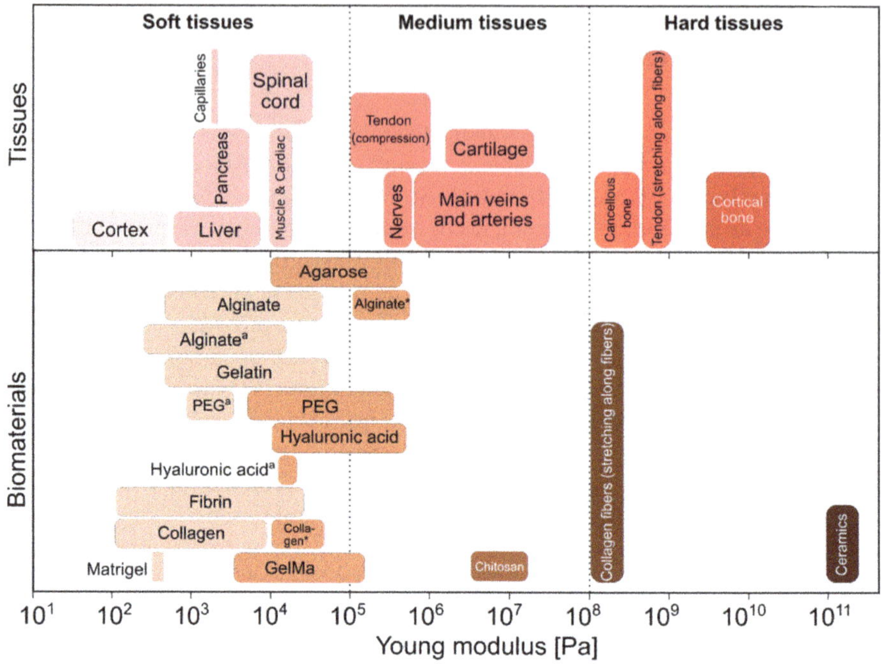

Fig. 2.3 Comparison of mechanical properties: tissues versus biomaterials. (*) Indicates hydrogels cross-linked under nonphysiological conditions; (a) refers to data obtained from microgels. Figure reproduced under license CC-BY-4.0 [75] (https://creativecommons.org/licenses/by/4.0/)

2.7 Advances in Tissue Anatomy Research

2.7.1 Bioimaging and Biophysical Techniques for Detailed Tissue Analysis

Recent advances in tissue anatomy research have been largely propelled by innovations in bioimaging and biophysical techniques that enable precise visualization and characterization of tissues at multiple scales. These technologies have transformed the understanding of tissue architecture, composition, and function, providing critical insights that inform the development of artificial tissues. Among the most impactful bioimaging modalities is multiphoton microscopy, which enables high-resolution, deep-tissue imaging without extensive tissue preparation or staining [78]. This technique exploits nonlinear optical effects to image living tissues in three dimensions, revealing cellular and extracellular matrix (ECM) organization with submicron resolution. Additionally, confocal laser scanning microscopy (CLSM) remains a cornerstone for detailed visualization of tissue components, allowing for optical sectioning and reconstruction of three-dimensional tissue structures. Both techniques facilitate the study of dynamic processes such as cell migration and matrix remodeling in situ.

Another significant development is super-resolution microscopy, which surpasses the diffraction limit of conventional light microscopy to resolve nanoscale features of tissues. Techniques such as STED (Stimulated Emission Depletion) and PALM (Photoactivated Localization Microscopy) enable visualization of molecular arrangements within cells and ECM, enhancing the understanding of tissue microarchitecture that is crucial for tissue engineering (see Fig. 2.4). Complementary to optical imaging, magnetic resonance imaging (MRI) and its variants, such as diffusion tensor imaging (DTI), allow for noninvasive, three-dimensional mapping of soft tissues in vivo. DTI provides insight into the orientation of fibrous tissues such as muscle and neural tracts, facilitating the reconstruction of tissue anisotropy and connectivity. Moreover, advancements in micro-computed tomography (micro-CT) have made it possible to visualize mineralized tissues like bone with micrometer-scale resolution, providing quantitative data on bone microstructure critical for designing biomimetic scaffolds. Biophysical characterization techniques have also evolved, offering quantitative measures of tissue mechanics, viscoelasticity, and cellular microenvironment properties. For instance, atomic force microscopy (AFM) has been widely used to probe the mechanical stiffness of tissues and ECM at the nanoscale, revealing heterogeneity in mechanical properties that guide cell behavior (see Fig. 2.4).

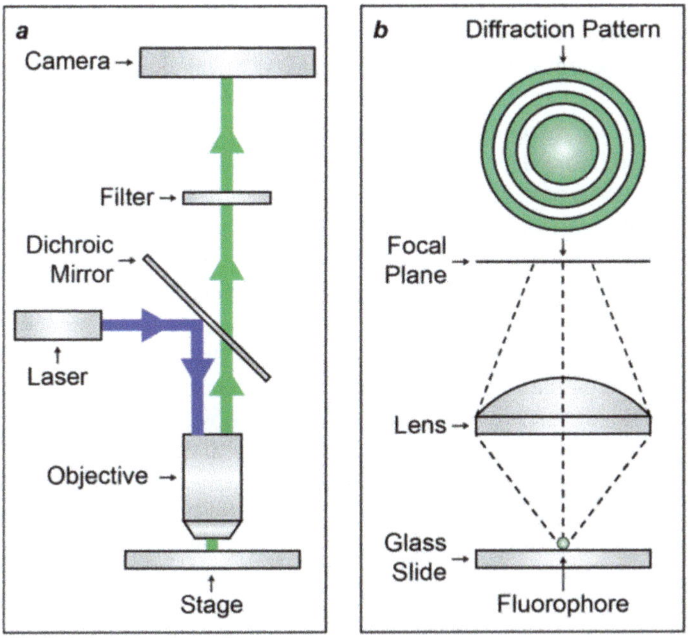

Fig. 2.4 Illustrates the key optical elements that make up a standard fluorescence microscope (**a**), alongside the characteristic Airy pattern (**b**) formed on the objective's focal plane when a single fluorophore emits light. Figure reproduced under license CC-BY-4.0 [79] (https://creativecommons.org/licenses/by/4.0/)

Similarly, optical tweezers and micropipette aspiration techniques enable manipulation and measurement of single-cell mechanical properties, enriching the understanding of mechanotransduction mechanisms in tissue formation. The integration of multi-modal imaging and biophysical analysis has culminated in powerful platforms that combine structural, mechanical, and biochemical data. These comprehensive approaches allow researchers to develop detailed tissue atlases and predictive models that inform scaffold design, cell seeding strategies, and bioreactor conditioning in artificial tissue engineering.

2.7.2 *Future Directions in Tissue Anatomy for Artificial Tissue Engineering*

The future of tissue anatomy research is poised to further enhance artificial tissue engineering through continued technological innovation and interdisciplinary integration. One promising direction is the advancement of in situ and real-time imaging techniques. Emerging modalities such as light-sheet fluorescence microscopy (LSFM) enable rapid volumetric imaging of living tissues with minimal phototoxicity, allowing longitudinal studies of tissue development and regeneration in engineered constructs. Furthermore, the convergence of tissue anatomy research with omics technologies (genomics, proteomics, metabolomics) offers a holistic understanding of tissue function at the molecular level. Spatial transcriptomics and proteomics facilitate mapping of gene and protein expression within tissue contexts, providing insight into cell heterogeneity, signaling pathways, and disease microenvironments that can be replicated in artificial tissues [80]. Integrating these molecular maps with anatomical imaging will enable precision engineering of tissue constructs tailored to specific physiological and pathological conditions. Artificial intelligence (AI) and machine learning (ML) are rapidly becoming instrumental in analyzing large and complex datasets generated by advanced imaging and biophysical studies. These computational tools can identify patterns, predict tissue behavior, and optimize scaffold design parameters, accelerating the translation of anatomical knowledge into functional tissue constructs [81]. For example, ML algorithms can aid in segmenting imaging data, quantifying tissue features, and modeling cell-ECM interactions under varying mechanical stimuli. Another emerging frontier is the development of biofabrication techniques that directly utilize detailed anatomical data to recreate native tissue architectures. High-resolution 3D bioprinting now incorporates microstructural features such as ECM fiber alignment and vascular network patterns, enabling fabrication of artificial tissues with improved biomimicry and functionality. Advances in biomaterials, including stimuli-responsive and smart hydrogels, complement these fabrication methods by providing dynamic microenvironments that support tissue remodeling and maturation. Finally, personalized medicine is expected to benefit greatly from these anatomical advancements. Patient-specific imaging combined with 3D printing and stem cell technologies will enable the production of customized artificial tissues and organs, reducing rejection risks and improving clinical outcomes [82]. Tissue anatomy research will thus play a critical role in bridging the gap between biological complexity and engineering solutions.

2.8 Conclusions

2.8.1 Summary of Tissue Anatomy and Its Relevance to Artificial Tissue Engineering

A comprehensive understanding of tissue anatomy is foundational to the advancement of artificial tissue engineering. Natural tissues are composed of diverse cells embedded within a highly specialized extracellular matrix (ECM), arranged into hierarchical structures that enable specific mechanical and physiological functions. The core classifications of tissues—epithelial, connective, muscle, and nervous—each serve unique roles in maintaining homeostasis, and their anatomical intricacies directly inform biomimetic strategies in tissue fabrication. Connective tissues, for example, display varied mechanical properties ranging from the pliability of areolar and adipose tissues to the rigidity of bone and cartilage. These tissues integrate cells such as fibroblasts or chondrocytes with ECM proteins like collagen, elastin, and glycosaminoglycans, forming a supportive network. Engineered analogues of these tissues, including synthetic bone and cartilage constructs, rely heavily on this anatomical blueprint for optimal integration and mechanical functionality in vivo. Muscle tissues—categorized into skeletal, cardiac, and smooth—are specialized for contractile functions. Their structure is defined by organized sarcomeres, actin-myosin interactions, and motor proteins that facilitate either voluntary or involuntary contractions. Artificial muscle constructs, such as bioactuators or engineered contractile tissues, have leveraged insights from this organization to replicate motion and force generation.

Nervous tissues, composed of neurons and glial cells, are responsible for processing and transmitting electrical impulses throughout the body. The unique anatomical features of the brain, spinal cord, and peripheral nerves, especially the organization of myelinated axons and synaptic networks, serve as templates for developing neural interfaces and regenerative strategies 6. Artificial neural tissue models aim to replicate these pathways for use in treating neurological injuries and diseases. Moreover, the biomechanical categorization of soft tissues into low, medium, and high stiffness further refines the approach to tissue engineering. For instance, tissues such as brain or lung are highly compliant, while tendons and ligaments exhibit substantial tensile strength. Understanding these distinctions is essential for matching material properties and ensuring mechanical compatibility with host tissues. Perhaps most significantly, comparative anatomy studies have revealed that artificial tissues often fall short in replicating the complex architecture, biomechanical behavior, and adaptive response of their natural counterparts. These limitations emphasize the need for anatomically precise design approaches in scaffold fabrication, cellular integration, and ECM synthesis. Although great strides have been made in mimicking gross structure, microstructural replication remains a major hurdle.

2.8.2 Future Prospects for Developing Artificial Tissues Based on Advanced Anatomical Understanding

Looking forward, continued progress in artificial tissue development is intricately linked to advances in anatomical science. Emerging imaging techniques such as multiphoton microscopy, super-resolution imaging, and diffusion tensor MRI have enabled detailed mapping of tissue microarchitecture in both static and dynamic states. These platforms allow real-time monitoring of cellular dynamics and tissue remodeling, greatly enhancing design feedback during scaffold optimization. Biophysical measurement tools like atomic force microscopy and micro-CT now permit nanoscale quantification of stiffness, porosity, and topography. These mechanical descriptors are essential for tailoring biomaterials that emulate the local mechanical environments of tissues, thus influencing stem cell differentiation and matrix deposition. For example, compliant scaffolds are being customized for brain-like tissues, whereas rigid scaffolds support osteogenic lineages.

Moreover, the integration of spatial transcriptomics and proteomics into tissue anatomy research provides unprecedented insight into molecular heterogeneity within tissues. This molecular mapping allows artificial tissues to be tuned not just structurally, but also biochemically, enhancing their physiological relevance. Artificial intelligence and machine learning further expand the potential of anatomical datasets by enabling complex pattern recognition, model prediction, and real-time adaptation during biofabrication. These technologies have already begun to influence automated segmentation of imaging data and optimization of bioprinting parameters.

On the fabrication front, 3D bioprinting has matured into a powerful platform for recapitulating natural tissue geometry. Innovations such as voxel-level printing, sacrificial bioinks for vascularization, and multi-material deposition now allow researchers to generate constructs with graded mechanical and biological properties, closely mimicking the heterogeneous nature of native tissues. Smart biomaterials, including thermoresponsive and shape-memory polymers, further allow engineered tissues to adapt in real time to changes in temperature, pH, or load. Ultimately, the convergence of anatomical insight with biotechnological tools will usher in a new generation of artificial tissues that are structurally, mechanically, and functionally indistinguishable from their natural counterparts. The vision of patient-specific tissue implants, informed by detailed anatomical and molecular datasets, is fast becoming a tangible reality. As this transformation unfolds, the field will benefit from ongoing collaborations among anatomists, material scientists, engineers, and clinicians who together strive to bring anatomical fidelity to the forefront of regenerative medicine.

References

1. McCormick RJ (1994) Structure and properties of tissues. In: Muscle foods, pp 25–62. https://doi.org/10.1007/978-1-4757-5933-4_2
2. Gupta S, Gupta V, Chanda A (2022) Biomechanical modeling of novel high expansion auxetic skin grafts. Int J Numer Method Biomed Eng 38:e3586
3. Chanda A, Gupta S (2025) Healthcare entrepreneurship and management. Routledge, Taylor & Francis Group
4. Biga LM et al (2019) Types of tissues
5. Lavker RM, Sun TT (2003) Epithelial stem cells: the eye provides a vision. Eye 17:937–942
6. Gupta S, Singh G, Chanda A (2021) Prediction of diabetic foot ulcer progression: a computational study. Biomed Phys Eng Express 7:065020
7. Singla R, Gupta S, Chanda A (2023) A computational fluid dynamics-based model for assessing rupture risk in cerebral arteries with varying aneurysm sizes. Math Comput Appl 28:90
8. Fisher JP (2007) Tissue engineering vascular grafts. Tissue Eng 439–452. https://doi.org/10.1201/9781420008333-33
9. Ellahi A, Gupta S, Bose D, Chanda A (2025) A high-fidelity biomechanical modeling framework for injury prediction during frontal car crash. Comput Methods Biomech Biomed Eng 28:13–24
10. Langer RS, Vacanti JP (1999) Tissue engineering: the challenges ahead. Sci Am 280:86–89
11. Yadav P et al (2025) Gelatin multiwalled carbon nanotube composite 3D printed semi biological mesh for abdominal hernia treatment. Chem Asian J 20:e202401136
12. Li Q, Tong Z, Mao H (2023) Microfluidic based organ-on-chips and biomedical application. Biosensors 13:436
13. Singh G, Yadav P, Chanda A (2024) Development of biofidelic skin simulants based on fresh cadaveric skin tests. Eur Burn J 5:454–463
14. Yadav P, Kamboj M, Das B (2024) Application of nanotechnology in antimicrobial coating on surgical instruments. Appl Nanotechnol Biomed Eng 150–168. https://doi.org/10.1201/9781003432661-9
15. Engler AJ, Sen S, Sweeney HL, Discher DE (2006) Matrix elasticity directs stem cell lineage specification. Cell 126:677–689
16. Verma S, Chanda A (2024) State-of-the-art of finite element modelling of the human spine to study the impact of vibrations: a review. Int J Comput Methods Eng Sci Mech 25:225–247
17. Watt FM, Hogan BLM (2000) Out of Eden: stem cells and their niches. Science 287:1427–1430
18. Verma S, Singh G, Chanda A (2023) A novel finite element model for the study of harmful vibrations on the aging spine. Computation 11:93
19. Verma S, Singh G, Chanda A (2024) Development of a computational framework for determination of detrimental vibrations on the human spine segments. Multiscale Sci Eng 6(1):48–56
20. Rozario T, DeSimone DW (2010) The extracellular matrix in development and morphogenesis: a dynamic view. Dev Biol 341:126–140
21. Schwertfeger KL, Cowman MK, Telmer PG, Turley EA, McCarthy JB (2015) Hyaluronan, inflammation, and breast cancer progression. Front Immunol 6:138645
22. Ingber DE (2008) Tensegrity and mechanotransduction. J Bodyw Mov Ther 12:198–200
23. Mukund K, Subramaniam S (2020) Skeletal muscle: a review of molecular structure and function, in health and disease. Wiley Interdiscip Rev Syst Biol Med 12:e1462
24. Srivastava D, Olson EN (1997) Knowing in your heart what's right. Trends Cell Biol 7:447–453
25. Gupta V, Chanda A (2021) Expansion potential of skin grafts with novel I-shaped auxetic incisions. Biomed Phys Eng Express 8:015016
26. Singh G, Chanda A (2024) Development and biomechanical testing of artificial surrogates for vaginal tissue. Adv Mater Process Technol. https://doi.org/10.1080/2374068X.2023.2198837
27. Morrison SJ, Spradling AC (2008) Stem cells and niches: mechanisms that promote stem cell maintenance throughout life. Cell 132:598–611

28. Chanda A (2018) Biomechanical modeling of human skin tissue surrogates. Biomimetics 3:18
29. Havis E, Duprez D (2020) EGR1 transcription factor is a multifaceted regulator of matrix production in tendons and other connective tissues. Int J Mol Sci 21(5):1664
30. Yang G, Rothrauff BB, Tuan RS (2013) Tendon and ligament regeneration and repair: clinical relevance and developmental paradigm. Birth Defects Res C Embryo Today 99:203
31. Chanda A, Gupta V, Gupta S (2024) Development and mechanical testing of auxetic incisions on human cadaveric skin, pp 89–99. https://doi.org/10.1007/978-981-97-4383-4_7
32. Gupta V, Singh G, Gupta S, Chanda A (2023) Expansion potential of auxetic prosthetic skin grafts: a review. Eng Res Express 5:022003
33. Gupta V, Singh G, Chanda A (2024) Modeling of metamaterial based incision patterns for generating high expansions in skin grafts. In: Lecture notes in mechanical engineering, pp 563–574. https://doi.org/10.1007/978-981-99-5919-8_51
34. Wang L, You X, Zhang L, Zhang C, Zou W (2022) Mechanical regulation of bone remodeling. Bone Res 101(10):1–15
35. Goodnough LT, Scott MG, Monk TG (1998) Oxygen carriers as blood substitutes: past, present, and future. Clin Orthop Relat Res 357:89–100
36. Singh G, Gupta V, Chanda A (2022) Mechanical characterization of rotating triangle shaped auxetic skin graft simulants. Fac Univ Ser Mech Eng
37. Singh G, Chanda A (2024) Biofidelic gallbladder tissue surrogates. Adv Mater Process Technol. https://doi.org/10.1080/2374068X.2023.2198835
38. Singh G, Gupta V, Chanda A (2022) Artificial skin with varying biomechanical properties. Mater Today Proc 62:3162–3166
39. McCuller C, Jessu R, Callahan AL (2023) Physiology, skeletal muscle. StatPearls
40. Bers DM (2002) Cardiac excitation-contraction coupling. Nature 415:198–205
41. Hill-Eubanks DC, Werner ME, Heppner TJ, Nelson MT (2011) Calcium signaling in smooth muscle. Cold Spring Harb Perspect Biol 3:a004549
42. Gupta V, Singh G, Chanda A (2023) Development of hierarchical auxetic skin graft simulants with high expansion potential. Biomed Eng Adv 5:100087
43. Jiang C et al (2022) Biomechanics of skin grafts: effect of pattern size, spacing and orientation. Eng Res Express 4:015006
44. Afazal M, Afreen S, Chanda A (2023) Computational modelling and analysis of hard tissue behavior around 0.5 mm and 0.85 mm platform switched abutment using 3D finite element analysis. Forces Mech 13:100243
45. Noble D (2002) Modeling the heart—from genes to cells to the whole organ. Science 295:1678–1682
46. Chhikara K, Gupta S, Bose D, Kataria C, Chanda A (2023) Development and trial of a multi-purpose customized orthosis for activities of daily living in patients with spinal cord injury. Prosthesis 5:467–479
47. Rothschild BM et al (2023) Design, manufacturing, and trial of a 3D printed customized finger splint for patients with rheumatoid arthritis. Rheumato 3:51–62
48. Vaughan CL, Davis BL, O'Connor JC (1999) Dynamics of human gait, 2nd edn, pp 16–17
49. Cvetkovic C et al (2014) Three-dimensionally printed biological machines powered by skeletal muscle. Proc Natl Acad Sci USA 111:10125–10130
50. Chanda A, Upchurch W (2018) Biomechanical modeling of wounded skin. J Compos Sci 2:69
51. Chhikara K, Gupta S, Chanda A (2022) Development of a novel foot orthosis for plantar pain reduction. Mater Today Proc 62:3532–3537
52. Shankar P et al (2022) A revolutionary breakthrough of bionanomaterials in tissue engineering and regenerative medicine, pp 399–441. https://doi.org/10.1016/B978-0-12-823915-5.00001-0
53. Chanda A, Chatterjee S, Gupta V (2020) Soft composite based hyperelastic model for anisotropic tissue characterization. J Compos Mater 54:4525–4534
54. Bose D, Gupta S, Chanda A (2025) Scalable direct manufacturing of a functional multipurpose wrist-hand orthosis using 3D printing. Ann 3D Print Med 17:100186
55. Chanda A, Ruchti T, Unnikrishnan V (2018) Computational modeling of wound suture: a review. IEEE Rev Biomed Eng 11:165–176

56. Singh G, Chanda A (2022) Biomechanical modeling of progressive wound healing: a computational study. Biomed Eng Adv 4:100055
57. Rashid B, Destrade M, Gilchrist MD (2014) Mechanical characterization of brain tissue in tension at dynamic strain rates. J Mech Behav Biomed Mater 33:43–54
58. Mattei G, Ahluwalia A (2016) Sample, testing and analysis variables affecting liver mechanical properties: a review. Acta Biomater 45:60–71
59. Geerligs M, Peters GWM, Ackermans PAJ, Oomens CWJ, Baaijens FPT (2008) Linear viscoelastic behavior of subcutaneous adipose tissue. Biorheology 45:677–688
60. Wilkie DR (1956) The mechanical properties of muscle. Br Med Bull 12:177–182
61. Li W (2015) Modelling methods for in vitro biomechanical properties of the skin: a review. Biomed Eng Lett 5:241–250
62. Mow VC, Guo XE (2002) Mechano-electrochemical properties of articular cartilage: their inhomogeneities and anisotropies. Annu Rev Biomed Eng 4:175–209
63. Provenzano PP, Vanderby R (2006) Collagen fibril morphology and organization: implications for force transmission in ligament and tendon. Matrix Biol 25:71–84
64. Espino DM, Shepherd DE, Hukins DW (2014) Viscoelastic properties of bovine knee joint articular cartilage: dependency on thickness and loading frequency. BMC Musculoskelet Disord 15:1–9
65. Chanda A, Flynn Z, Unnikrishnan V (2018) Biomechanical characterization of normal and prolapsed vaginal tissue surrogates. J Mech Med Biol 18. https://doi.org/10.1142/S0219519417501007
66. Singh G, Chanda A (2024) Finite element modeling of diabetic foot: a state-of-the-art review. Eng Res Express 6:012507
67. Gupta V, Chanda A (2024) Mechanical characterization of alternating slit, I-shaped and rotating triangle based auxetic skin graft phantoms. Mech Adv Mater Struct. https://doi.org/10.1080/15376494.2023.2250782
68. Del Bakhshayesh AR et al (2019) An overview of advanced biocompatible and biomimetic materials for creation of replacement structures in the musculoskeletal systems: focusing on cartilage tissue engineering. J Biol Eng 13(1):1–21
69. Alkaron W, Almansoori A, Balázsi C, Balázsi K (2024) A critical review of natural and synthetic polymer-based biological apatite composites for bone tissue engineering. J Compos Sci 8:523
70. Reddy MSB, Ponnamma D, Choudhary R, Sadasivuni KK (2021) A comparative review of natural and synthetic biopolymer composite scaffolds. Polymers (Basel) 13:1105
71. Echeverria Molina MI, Malollari KG, Komvopoulos K (2021) Design challenges in polymeric scaffolds for tissue engineering. Front Bioeng Biotechnol 9:617141
72. Liu S et al (2023) Biomimetic natural biomaterials for tissue engineering and regenerative medicine: new biosynthesis methods, recent advances, and emerging applications. Mil Med Res 10(1):1–30
73. Chanda A, Unnikrishnan V, Flynn Z, Lackey K (2017) Experimental study on tissue phantoms to understand the effect of injury and suturing on human skin mechanical properties. Proc Inst Mech Eng Part H J Eng Med 231:80–91
74. Gupta V, Chanda A (2023) Biomechanical modelling of hierarchical metamaterials for skin grafting. In: Materials horizons: from nature to nanomaterials (part F1471), pp 71–83
75. Rojek KO, Ćwiklińska M, Kuczak J, Guzowski J (2022) Microfluidic formulation of topological hydrogels for microtissue engineering. Chem Rev 122:16839–16909
76. Andorko JI, Christopher, Jewell M, Jewell CM (2017) Designing biomaterials with immunomodulatory properties for tissue engineering and regenerative medicine. Bioeng Transl Med 2:139–155
77. Tortorici M, Petersen A, Duda GN, Checa S (2022) The degradation of synthetic polymeric scaffolds with strut-like architecture influences the mechanics-dependent repair process of an osteochondral defect in silico. Front Bioeng Biotechnol 10:846665
78. Zipfel WR, Williams RM, Webb WW (2003) Nonlinear magic: multiphoton microscopy in the biosciences. Nat Biotechnol 21:1369–1377

79. Zhang Y, Zheng Y, Tomassini A, Singh AK, Raymo FM (2023) Photoactivatable BODIPYs for live-cell PALM. Molecules 28:2447
80. Ståhl PL et al (2016) Visualization and analysis of gene expression in tissue sections by spatial transcriptomics. Science 353:78–82
81. Esteva A et al (2019) A guide to deep learning in healthcare. Nat Med 25:24–29
82. Lavik E, Langer R (2004) Tissue engineering: current state and perspectives. Appl Microbiol Biotechnol 65:1–8

Chapter 3
Imaging of Tissues

3.1 Introduction

The area of tissue engineering is constantly changing due to multidisciplinary research employing cutting-edge technologies from engineering, molecular biology, synthetic chemistry, pharmaceutics, and medicine, among other disciplines. Tissue engineering is now fast moving toward therapeutic applications and has advanced beyond in vitro and animal research as a result. Tissue engineering technology advances toward nanoscale material creation techniques as it develops. Therefore, tissue engineers want adaptable imaging techniques that can track not only morphological but also functional and molecular information to evaluate improved tissue engineering applications. Many tissue engineering investigations proceed with utilizing the use of traditional instruments, such as histology procedures, which offer valuable but constrained information, particularly when it comes to in vivo preclinical and clinical approaches [1]. Because the samples must be destroyed in order to visualize tissue-engineered constructions using these traditional techniques, longitudinal three-dimensional (3D) volumetric measurement is severely constrained. Additionally, histology needs statistical analysis to account for discrepancies in experimental results from different samples and at different times due to destructive methods and limited views within the confined volume. Tissue engineers have access to a wide range of sophisticated imaging methods, and more and more current tissue engineering research efforts are being conducted to investigate the uses of several sophisticated imaging modalities [2–4]. The limitations of traditional instruments can be overcome by using advanced imaging techniques to monitor tissue-engineered constructions noninvasively, longitudinally, and consistently.

Using safe, quantitative, and non-invasive monitoring, the optimal imaging tool for tissue engineering must be relevant to both human and animal research at the subcellular level. The optimal imaging technique needs to be able to resolve signals at the subcellular scale and penetrate through the entire body in order to support all the various applications. Furthermore, the imaging device should preferably provide

A. Chanda and D. Sharma, *Handbook of Artificial Tissues, Biofabrication and Bioprinting, Volume I*, Biomedical Materials for Multi-functional Applications,
https://doi.org/10.1007/978-981-92-1307-8_3

contrast in order to provide all relevant data on morphological, physiological, and molecular alterations. Nevertheless, there isn't really a single imaging modality that can be used for all tissue-engineered construct applications and information. The physical interaction between an internal or external energy source (such as electromagnetic waves, pressure waves, etc.) and the object being imaged (such as tissues, organs, cells, nanoparticles, molecules, etc.) is the foundation of all medical imaging systems available for tissue engineering; the imaging systems detect the energy change transmitted from the object to form an image. Thus, the intensity and wavelength of energy sources, as well as the features of the imaging system, define certain aspects of medical imaging techniques, including spatial and temporal resolution, penetration depth, appropriate endogenous and exogenous contrast agents, safety, and cost [5]. As a result, each imaging approach has a unique set of applications and information depending on its unique qualities. Consequently, tissue engineers should choose the best instrument from diverse imaging modalities based on the needs of the tissue engineering investigations. The objective of this chapter is to outline the biomedical imaging techniques that may be used to evaluate tissue engineering applications and to give tissue engineers standards and information for choosing the most effective imaging approaches. The most recent trends of their applications in recent tissue engineering studies will be the main focus of this discussion, which will cover commonly used biomedical imaging modalities such as X-ray and computed tomography (CT), positron emission tomography (PET), and single photon emission computed tomography (SPECT), magnetic resonance imaging (MRI), ultrasound imaging, optical imaging, emerging techniques, and multimodal imaging [6–8].

3.2 Tissue Engineering Imaging Approaches

3.2.1 X-Ray/CT

Since its inception, radiographic imaging, which includes CT and X-ray imaging, has served as the primary diagnostic technique. Its usage has grown quickly because of its exceptional contrast and spatial resolution for displaying anatomy, particularly bone structure. Since X-ray energy is far more concentrated than light energy and can pass through the human body, it serves as the energy source for radiographic imaging [9]. The attenuation of the projected X-ray beam is measured to produce images from CT and X-ray imaging. Clinical techniques are made possible by the exceptional penetration depth of CT and X-ray imaging, which are made possible by the high level of the imaging energy source. X-ray radiation, on the other hand, is ionizing and can harm materials or tissue. Furthermore, the contrast between soft tissues is not as great as that of bone, despite the fact that CT and X-ray imaging are effective methods for imaging bone. Additionally, compared to other molecular imaging methods, contrast agents are still scarce, despite some researchers' exploration of functional and molecular imaging using CT and X-ray imaging. In bone and tissue engineering research, CT and micro-CT imaging methods are essential, especially for assessing scaffold integration and bone regeneration. These X-ray-based techniques are useful for evaluating treatments meant to repair bone abnormalities because they enable researchers to non-invasively track changes in bone shape, mineralization, and vascularization over time [10–12]. Because bone absorbs a lot of X-rays, CT, and X-ray imaging are good ways to see new bone deposition. Understanding how well these scaffolds assist bone regeneration requires being able to record bone development and integration into different porous scaffold materials. For example, CT imaging has provided insight into the intricate processes of mineral deposition at the organic-mineral interface by displaying the development of bone mineralization at various distances from the scaffold interface. Researchers can better understand how bone grows and interacts with scaffolds by watching these stages, which is essential for creating successful treatments [13–15].

Micro-CT is often utilized in both in vitro and in vivo situations because of its high-resolution capabilities. For instance, scaffolds implanted with human mesenchymal stem cells have had their bone mineralization conditions optimized through the use of micro-CT (see Fig. 3.1). This approach was used by Olaret et al. to characterize the engineered scaffolds with biomedical applications. They found that extracting the hydrogel, a natural polymer, from the polypropylene framework presented some challenges. Due to the differing water affinities of the polymers, the contrast between them was enhanced by selectively staining the hydrogel with an aqueous silver nitrate solution [13, 16, 17].

Scaffolds composed of different materials and subjected to static or perfused medium flow conditions have been analyzed by researchers using micro-CT. The best culture conditions to encourage osteogenesis and improve bone formation may be found with the use of this imaging technology, which offers comprehensive insights into the spatial distribution and interconnectedness of bone growth inside the scaffold. Researchers may adjust scaffold materials and culture conditions to promote bone repair and regeneration by visualizing the distribution of bones within scaffolds [18]. The requirement for contrast chemicals in CT imaging is a problem, particularly for scaffolds with intricate architecture. To improve visibility in micro- or nano-CT imaging, scaffolds are frequently coated with hexabrix, a frequently used contrast agent. Hexabrix, for example, has been utilized to image chondrocyte-seeded silk fibroin scaffolds, evaluate proteoglycan synthesis, and determine if the scaffold is suitable for cartilage tissue engineering. However, the contrast compounds also have limitations affecting the overall performance of the system. For instance, phosphotungstic acid (PTA) cannot completely cover every scaffold surface, which could result in misleading blank gaps on CT scans. These imaging distortions may misrepresent the density or composition of the scaffold, which can have an impact on how data is interpreted. While previous depth-limited approaches may misread scaffold composition due to incomplete ECM coverage, nano-CT, an even more precise imaging technology, might assist overcome these limitations by precisely identifying extracellular matrix (ECM) deposition surrounding scaffold peripheries [19–21].

Another cutting-edge technique that tackles certain CT imaging issues is X-ray phase-contrast micro-CT imaging. Without the use of potentially harmful contrast

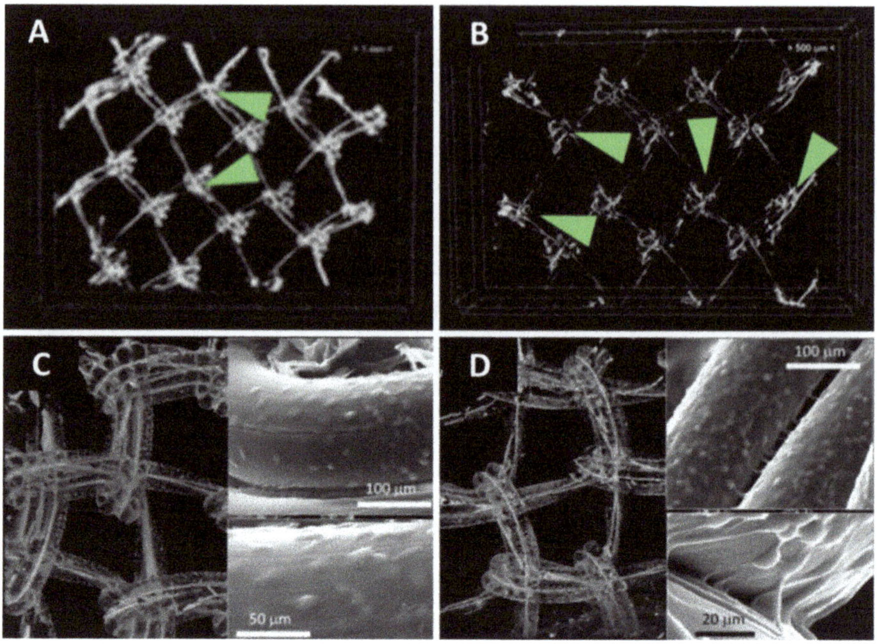

Fig. 3.1 Micro-CT images captured post-coating revealing: **a** hydrogel coating applied to a polypropylene mesh after seven days of uniaxial tension testing in an acellular environment; **b** micro-CT scans taken; **c** one-day post-cell seeding; and **d** seven days post-cell seeding. Figure reproduced under license CC-BY-4.0 [13] (https://creativecommons.org/licenses/by/4.0/)

chemicals, this method improves the visibility of light components frequently present in soft tissues. Cell-seeded poly(lactic-co-glycolic) acid (PLGA) scaffolds have been seen using phase-contrast imaging, which tracks how cells alter the scaffold over time. Phase-contrast micro-CT offers an option for investigating scaffolds in a manner that more truly represents tissue integration and alteration, which is essential for evaluating scaffold biocompatibility and degradation since traditional X-ray imaging has limited soft-tissue contrast [22–24]. Micro-CT is also useful for observing the vasculature inside tissue-engineered structures. Researchers can improve the visibility of the vascular network within scaffold structures in ex vivo samples by employing radiopaque chemicals like Microfil or barium sulfate. To evaluate vascularization, for instance, research has employed Microfil-enhanced micro-CT to examine vascular structures inside a scaffold made of hydroxyapatite and tricalcium phosphate in conjunction with an arteriovenous loop. In contrast to conventional 2D histology techniques, the 3D pictures produced by micro-CT offer comprehensive views of the vascular architecture within the scaffold, enabling precise quantification. Notwithstanding its advantages, micro-CT has resolution limits, and insufficient vessel filling with contrast agents may result in inaccurate vascular measurement. Because vessels in close proximity might merge, micro-CT may occasionally overestimate vessel sizes, which can skew results. CT, micro-CT, and phase-contrast imaging methods are essential for non-invasively examining scaffold integration and bone regeneration in tissue engineering. To create successful bone and tissue engineering treatments, these imaging techniques offer vital information on scaffold optimization, tissue compatibility, and vascularization. Researchers can more accurately evaluate scaffold performance and enhance treatment results for bone defect repairs and tissue engineering applications by selecting the appropriate imaging technology and being aware of its limits [25–28].

3.2.2 Nuclear Medicine (PET/SPECT)

A potent diagnostic technique for assessing the functional and molecular information of the imaged target is nuclear medicine, which encompasses PET and SPECT. The use of radioactive substances, which can localize in certain organs or tissues based on their biochemical or physiological characteristics, is the basic idea behind PET/SPECT imaging. Nuclear imaging offers the ability to track functional processes since some substances of biological relevance may be radiolabeled. PET and SPECT are the primary molecular imaging methods with the highest sensitivity among the many isotopes available as contrast agents in biomedical imaging modalities for full-body imaging. Furthermore, there are a number of isotopes that may be used as contrast agents for nuclear medicine imaging methods like PET and SPECT, which have extremely high sensitivity [29–31]. But like X-ray and CT, PET and SPECT are ionizing since they rely on the detection of gamma rays from the isotopes. Tissue-engineered structures cannot be seen at the sub-millimeter level due to the high cost of nuclear imaging modalities and the low spatial and temporal resolution of nuclear medicine. In tissue engineering and regenerative medicine, PET and SPECT imaging are useful technologies that provide non-invasive ways to track the incorporation of scaffolds in injury models and stem cell treatments. These imaging methods are helpful in understanding cellular function, location, and metabolic activity, which is measured by fluorodeoxyglucose (18F-FDG) absorption by following stem and progenitor cells in vivo. While PET and SPECT have also been used to track stem cells within bone scaffolds, FDG-PET has shown promise in assessing functional recovery in infarcted regions after cell distribution in heart damage models. When combined with CT imaging, these methods offer information on the scaffold's structural integration into the tissue as well as cellular viability. Histology confirms the functional integrity of endothelial cells within vascular networks.

In the pursuit of osteogenesis in bone abnormalities, PET imaging has proven especially helpful. PET has shown improved bone production and vascularization by the use of genetically modified bone marrow-derived mesenchymal stem cells (MSCs) that produce vascular endothelial growth factor (VEGF) and bone morphogenetic protein (BMP2). SPECT has also been used to follow adipose-derived stem cells transfected with BMP2 and VEGF for bone restoration, allowing evaluations of osteogenic capacity and scaffold integration over time [32–35]. For instance, in order to maximize scaffold conditions for sustained growth factor dispersion and facilitate efficient healing, BMP2 tagged with 125I was monitored for 28 days. Researchers can adjust scaffold designs for improved therapeutic results by tracking growth factor release within tissue scaffolds. The use of PET and SPECT in tissue engineering has been further expanded by the development of sophisticated contrast agents that target certain biological markers. For instance, angiogenesis may be seen using probes that target the angiogenesis marker avb3 integrin. This is essential for the healing of vascularized tissue. In mouse models, biodegradable nanoprobes functionalized with RGD peptides and tagged with radio halogen 76Br exhibited preferential absorption in ischemic tissue, indicating their potential for non-invasive angiogenesis monitoring in scaffold and cell therapy applications. In tracking stem cell activity, scaffold integration, and growth factor release in regenerative medicine requires the use of PET and SPECT imaging. Incorporating sophisticated contrast agents also makes it possible to image angiogenesis precisely, providing real-time information that is essential for developing tissue-engineering applications and improving cell-based treatments [36–39].

Contrast chemicals that target certain biological pathways within the body have been created for PET and SPECT imaging. Probes that are specific to avb3, a biological marker of angiogenesis, have been created for noninvasive angiogenesis imaging in tissue engineering applications. Almutairi et al. [32] created one example of these biodegradable probes, which are made up of eight branches that are functionalized at the ends of polymer chains with the radiohalogen 76Br and the targeting peptide RGD. In an in vivo model of hindlimb ischemia in mice, the nanoprobes demonstrated a high selective uptake in angiogenesis-related muscles. These contrast compounds may be used to track the degree of related angiogenesis in conjunction with tissue-engineered scaffolds and cell treatments [40–43].

3.3 Imaging with Magnetic Resonance

MRI's deep penetration and safety profile make it a popular imaging tool in preclinical and clinical settings. In order to make use of the magnetic characteristics of atoms, which spin at a certain Larmor frequency depending on their surroundings, MRI aligns nuclei (mostly hydrogen ^{1}H) within a magnetic field (1.5–10 T). MRI visualizes proton density or T1 and T2 relaxation durations by applying and detecting radiofrequency (RF) pulses that produce signals that change depending on the characteristics of the tissue. With its great spatial resolution (~ 100 μm) and even stronger fields (7–9 T), micro-MRI allows for comprehensive tissue imaging for applications like tissue engineering. Because of its great contrast between soft tissues, MRI is very useful for imaging anatomy. Furthermore, contrast agents—usually iron oxide or gadolinium-based nanoparticles—can improve vision even further by facilitating tracking and contrast. These substances make MRI a potent modality for a variety of imaging requirements by enabling it to transmit anatomical, functional, and even cellular information [44–48]. However, MRI has limited sensitivity to molecular interactions and only provides a limited selection of molecular probes, despite its superiority in structural and some functional imaging. Because of this drawback, MRI is less useful for molecular imaging than other techniques created specifically for that use. As a result, while MRI is very useful in many situations, it might not be the best option for applications that need close observation of molecular interactions. In vitro and in vivo, MRI can visualize and evaluate tissue-engineered structures without the need of external contrast agents due to its improved capacity to discern soft tissue contrast. The evaluation of tissue-engineered constructions has been shown in a number of in vitro MRI investigations. For example, measured MR relaxation durations (T1, T2) and diffusion coefficients have been used to evaluate the composition of bladder acellular matrix-based scaffolds. After hydrogel has been incorporated into cartilage, MRI has also been utilized to assess intermediary adhesive layers using changes in the scaffolds' magnetization relaxation times [49–52]. Furthermore, it was shown in vitro that variations in MR characteristics were connected with cell activities, like chondrocyte development and mesenchymal stem cell differentiation in the gels. The resorption of adipose tissue-engineered structures was longitudinally observed in vivo using MRI since fat tissues have a short T1 relaxation period. Additionally, utilizing quantitative T2 mapping, the healing of articular cartilage in a rabbit osteochondral lesion model was tracked over time following thrombin peptide (TP)-508 therapy. Because MRI can follow cell and scaffold structures inside tissues noninvasively, it is widely employed in tissue engineering. Figure 3.2 shows the anatomical data collected using the WS-bSSFP sequence after the biomaterials were implanted in rats. One-week post-implantation, all defects filled with biomaterials were distinctly visible as hyper-intense regions within the bone marrow, contrasting with the hypo-intense appearance of healthy bone (indicated by arrows in Fig. 3.2a). Over time, the hyper-intense signal from defects filled with Matrix-HA and Matrix-HA-Fuco biomaterials gradually diminished, whereas the signal from the defect containing Matrix-Fuco remained detectable for up to five weeks after implantation [53–56].

However, it can be difficult to monitor individual cells with MRI because there may not be enough contrast between the cells and the surrounding tissues. Magnetic compounds such as gadolinium and superparamagnetic iron oxide nanoparticles (SPIONs) are commonly used to improve vision. These substances enhance imaging contrast and make it possible to see different cell types in vivo or within scaffolds, including mesenchymal stem cells, astrocytes, and chondrocytes. To illustrate how these improvements may efficiently track cell localization in a real organism, gadolinium-labeled endothelial progenitor cells were monitored after implantation in an ischemia rat model [57]. Additionally, scaffolds are labeled with magnetic materials to aid in visualizing the shape and structure of implanted biomaterials. This is especially helpful in bone tissue engineering, where low hydrogen content and rapid T2 relaxation durations make replacements like calcium phosphate cements difficult to image. These restrictions are removed by combining iron oxide particles with gadolinium or single-walled carbon nanotubes, which enables these bone replacements to be distinguished from natural bone formations. In one instance, collagen scaffolds were labeled with SPIONs, allowing for subcutaneous in vivo monitoring of their breakdown. Hydrogel filaments based on gadolinium and SPIO have also

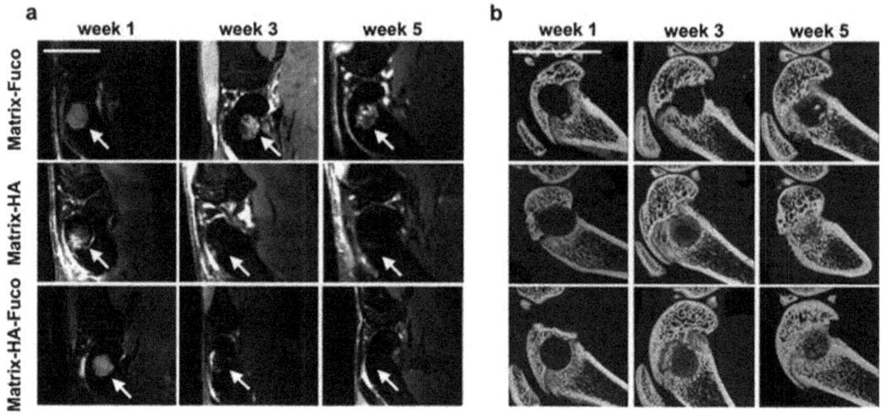

Fig. 3.2 **a** 3D WS-bSSFP in vivo representative images; **b** representative 2D images of the median region from ex vivo micro-CT 3D reconstructions of femoral condyles obtained 1, 3, and 5 weeks after implanting Matrix-Fuco, Matrix-HA, and Matrix-HA-Fuco matrices (indicated by arrows). Figure reproduced under license CC-BY-4.0 [56] (https://creativecommons.org/licenses/by/4.0/)

been created for MRI imaging, which helps with treatments like cerebral aneurysm embolization by providing a clear vision of the implant [58]. By using a method known as magnetic resonance elastography (MRE), MRI may evaluate mechanical characteristics such as stiffness and elasticity in addition to structural imaging. MRE analyzes mechanical properties such as the shear elastic modulus, which reflects the connection between stress and strain in tissues, using low-frequency shear waves produced by an acoustic actuator. Because it allows for the non-invasive monitoring of characteristics necessary for functioning tissue, this use is very beneficial in tissue engineering. MRE has been used in studies to discern developmental phases in engineered fat and follow the osteogenic and adipogenic advances of mesenchymal stem cell-based constructs in vivo, which was not possible with T2-weighted MRI alone. MRI has become an essential tool in clinical research, particularly in tissue engineering, due to its capacity to offer comprehensive morphological, functional, and molecular data without requiring invasive procedures. MRI has been used to track tissue-engineered constructions for therapeutic applications, including pulmonary valves, in order to identify problems like wall thickening that might be a sign of graft failure. By recording the dynamic contrast as new blood vessels develop inside the scaffold, MRI has also been used to evaluate neovascularization in bone substitutes for maxillary sinus augmentation. Ultimately, MRI's rising importance in regenerative medicine and clinical applications is supported by the substantial benefits it provides for tracking cell and scaffold integration, evaluating mechanical qualities, and monitoring vascularization in tissue engineering [59, 60].

3.4 Ultrasound Imaging

With benefits including biocompatibility, high temporal resolution, customizable penetration depth, mobility, and affordability, ultrasound imaging is a commonly used diagnostic technique. In order to change depth and resolution for applications ranging from scaffold imaging to clinical research, ultrasonic waves are sent via a transducer, which then receives the reflected waves from tissues [61]. Ultrasound imaging contrast is based on variations in acoustic impedance, which are influenced by bulk modulus and tissue density. Because of this, tissue-engineered constructions may have their mechanical and structural characteristics captured by ultrasonography in both laboratory and clinical contexts. Grayscale ultrasonic scans, for instance, have been used to measure the amount of collagen in fibrin-based structures and monitor the mineralization of collagen hydrogels. Additionally, by examining sound speed and attenuation, ultrasonography has tracked the breakdown in hydrogels encapsulated in chondrocytes [62]. Even more precise information is provided by high-frequency ultrasonic microscopy, which enables scientists to study the mechanical characteristics of synthetic cartilage in animal models following transplantation. Three-dimensional reconstructions of a human knee generated using the combined speed of sound (SOS) and reflection images are illustrated in Fig. 3.3. In the coronal view, the vastus and lateral collateral ligament exhibit the expected high SOS on the left side of the image. The trabecular bone, characterized by a lower apparent SOS, is enclosed by high-speed cortical bone and periosteum. The reduced SOS within the trabecular bone may suggest the influence of the slow Biot compressional wave or represent an "effective" SOS, reflecting the averaged SOS of the bone matrix and the fluid within the trabecular structure [62].

When using bioresorbable scaffold implants to evaluate the course of atherosclerosis at coronary bifurcations, intravascular ultrasonography has been shown to be

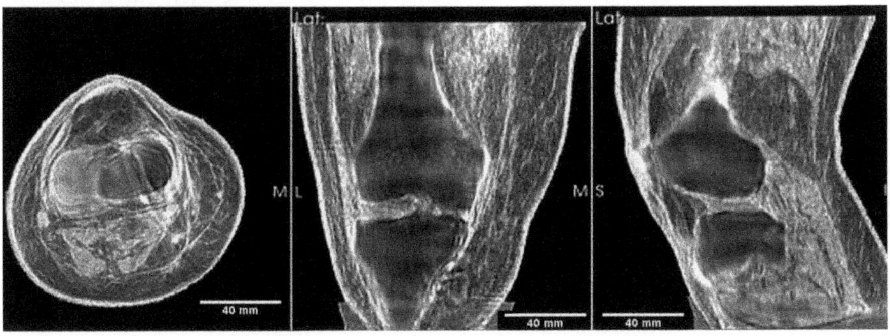

Fig. 3.3 Axial, coronal, and sagittal images from a 3D speed of sound (SOS) map generated through transmission ultrasonography were combined with a reflection image to create a fused representation of a fully developed human knee. This visualization highlights the three-dimensional nature of the reconstruction. The articular cartilage in the tibiofemoral region is clearly visible. Figure reproduced under license CC-BY-4.0 [62] (https://creativecommons.org/licenses/by/4.0/)

useful in clinical settings [63]. Additionally, ultrasound aids in the clinical assessment of autologous tissue-engineered vascular grafts, proving their efficacy and durability as arteriovenous shunts in patients with end-stage renal illness. All things considered, ultrasonography plays a crucial role in tissue engineering for noninvasively tracking mechanical and structural properties as well as implant integration over time. When it comes to tracking tissue-engineered vascular grafts and other structures, ultrasound imaging is essential, especially when evaluating the grafts long-term integration and endurance. Ultrasound imaging is used to monitor the durability of designed vascular grafts in hemodialysis patients, especially to search for indications of aneurysm development or wall degeneration. This capacity is essential for maintaining patient safety and long-term transplant function [64]. Doppler ultrasonography has been used in conjunction with air bubble injection to assess tissue-engineered heart valves. This technique ensures efficient volume replenishment in flow-loop bioreactors, which aids in verifying appropriate valve performance, particularly in models based on tubular leaflet designs. Doppler ultrasonography makes it possible to precisely monitor valve function and make necessary real-time modifications by producing a visual depiction of blood flow [65].

Furthermore, the use of ultrasonography in describing tissue-engineered vascular networks has increased due to the introduction of microbubbles into extracellular matrix scaffolds. Using this method, ultrasonography may assess critical features such microvessel volumes and diameters, flow rates, and 3D vessel design [66]. Additionally, microbubbles aid in the differentiation of vascular structures from matrix components, improving the precision and detail of ultrasonic evaluations in intricate scaffolds. Because it gives a clear picture of scaffold performance and vascularization in real-time, this feature is especially helpful for comprehending the structure and integration of designed vascular networks [67]. These uses collectively highlight the value and adaptability of ultrasound in tissue engineering. Ultrasound greatly advances clinical and preclinical studies in regenerative medicine by facilitating non-invasive and comprehensive monitoring of graft integrity, valve function, and vascular scaffold integration. Its application is further expanded by its usage in Doppler and microbubble-enhanced imaging techniques, which makes it a crucial instrument for evaluating created tissues in both clinical and research contexts.

3.5 Optical Imaging

Tissue engineering makes extensive use of optical imaging, particularly through optical and fluorescence microscopy, because of its high sensitivity and superior spatial resolution. These imaging techniques are especially well-suited for research projects that seek to collect cellular and molecular data because they make it easier to employ different biomarkers to track intracellular signaling and cellular interactions. However, photon scattering frequently restricts optical imaging's efficacy and prevents it from imaging deeper tissues. Thus, optical microscopy has mostly been limited to in vitro research, in vivo skin model inspections, and ex vivo confirmations like histology [68]. Notwithstanding these difficulties, optical microscopy is still a useful technique for examining and evaluating the molecular functioning of tissue-engineered structures. Excellent spatial resolution, a variety of exogenous and endogenous contrast agents, and great specificity are some of its strengths. This makes it possible for scientists to examine the functions of matrix-embedded cells in engineered tissues and to differentiate between matrix and matrix-embedded cells [69]. Recent developments have greatly enhanced optical imaging's capabilities, especially in two-photon and multiphoton fluorescence microscopy. Through multiphoton absorption, these methods lessen background signals and optical attenuation, allowing for depth-resolved imaging with penetration depths of up to 500 mm. Even in bioreactor environments, this improved imaging capacity enables researchers to see the architecture of synthetic tissues and polymer gels at different depths [70]. Additionally, mesenchymal stem cells placed in a variety of settings, including rat skin, silk, chitosan, and acellular scaffolds, have been successfully monitored using these sophisticated fluorescence imaging methods. Two-photon fluorescence microscopy and similar techniques represent a major advancement in tissue engineering by offering comprehensive insights into the cellular milieu and the functions of created tissues.

Chalal et al. [71] presented a study of how optical imaging may help create novel biomaterials and treatment approaches, which will ultimately advance the area of regenerative medicine. Because of its capacity to enter deeper into tissues while displaying minimal optical absorption, macroscopic imaging techniques employing near-infrared (NIR) fluorescence probes are increasing in importance in the area of tissue engineering. This feature enables scientists to efficiently track biological processes in vivo across long stretches of time. Furthermore, NIR-targeted probes have made it easier to see mineralization over time in tissue-engineered osteogenic structures, demonstrating how NIR fluorescence imaging may provide information about tissue growth and repair. NIR fluorescence imaging has several benefits, yet there are still issues with spatial resolution. To evaluate the penetration depth advantage of NIR-II phosphorescence, Yoon et al. [72] conducted in vitro imaging using a sample coated with 1% intralipid to simulate real tissue. In Fig. 3.4, a 5 mm thick intralipid layer, the phosphorescent nanotubes achieved a signal-to-noise ratio of approximately 15.6, compared to 1.9 for fluorescent nanorods. For in vivo analysis, the tumor's surrounding skin was removed, and nanotubes were injected intratumorally at a depth of 5 mm. NIR-II phosphorescence imaging was then performed. Mice injected with PEG-coated nanorods showed very faint signals in the tumor region, whereas those injected with nanotubes exhibited a clear NIR-II signal [72].

In macroscopic fluorescent imaging, the phenomena of optical scattering can reduce picture quality, making it more challenging to acquire precise depth-resolved evaluations. The necessity for other imaging modalities that can offer both depth and resolution is highlighted by this constraint [73]. OCT, or optical coherence tomography, has become an alternative substitute for tissue engineering and other uses. OCT records reflected signals from the sample and compares them to a reference

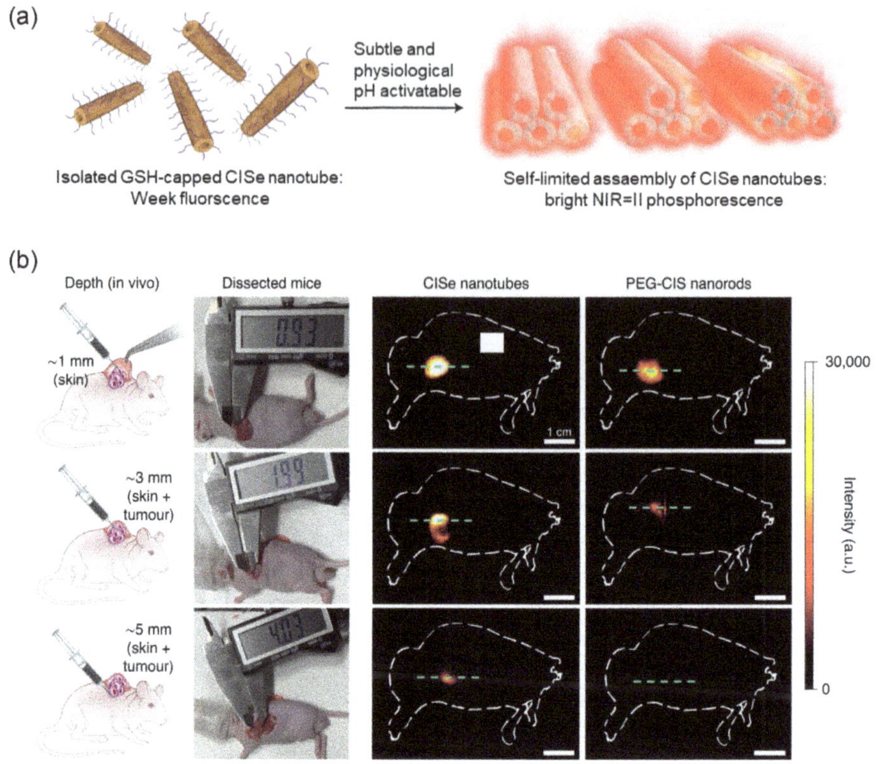

Fig. 3.4 **a** Schematic illustration of the assembly of the nanotubes; **b** imaging signal attenuation test conducted on tumor-bearing mice. Figure reproduced under license CC-BY-4.0 [72] (https://creativecommons.org/licenses/by/4.0/)

signal using the interference and coherence approaches. OCT may provide anatomical information with a penetration depth of less than a millimetre, which links OCT more to optical scattering than to fluorescence or absorption. OCT has been shown in studies to be able to assess pore size and volume porosity in macroporous hydrogel scaffolds without causing any damage. Because it eliminates the need for sample sectioning and staining, which are frequently necessary in fluorescence microscopy, such non-invasive imaging is especially useful for longitudinal investigations that track the growth of tissue-engineered skin over time. OCT has also been used in clinical settings since it is non-invasive, especially in intravascular imaging. Notably, OCT has been used to see implanted vascular scaffolds and to image the development of neotima in patients over a period of four years [74].

Another cutting-edge optical imaging method is bioluminescence imaging, which uses an internal light source created when luciferase oxidizes luciferin in the presence of oxygen and ATP. Bioluminescence imaging makes it possible to introduce different luciferase reporters inside cells, in contrast to conventional optical imaging techniques that need external light sources. Real-time metabolic activity monitoring is therefore possible by delivering these cells into living beings and integrating them into tissue-engineered constructions. External photon detectors, which have great sensitivity and minimal background noise, capture the light released by metabolically active cells, improving measurement accuracy. Because of this characteristic, bioluminescence imaging is a great tool for long-term in vivo investigations of cellular data in tiny animal models, where conventional imaging methods might not be sufficient [75]. Bioluminescence imaging has been shown to be effective in evaluating a number of biological processes, including the osteogenic differentiation and proliferation of luciferase-labeled mesenchymal stem cells in scaffolds over a period of weeks. Furthermore, the adaptability of this imaging technique has been demonstrated by scientists who have used hypoxia-responsive elements connected to luciferase to observe hypoxia in tissue-engineered scaffolds successfully [76]. Bioluminescence imaging has drawbacks despite its many benefits. Applications requiring precise three-dimensional reconstruction, quantitative analysis, or high spatial resolution (beyond the millimetre level) are not appropriate for it. Furthermore, the technique's use in clinical settings is restricted due to the safety of bioluminescent genes. Therefore, even though macroscopic visualization techniques like OCT, bioluminescence imaging, and NIR fluorescence provide useful tools for developing tissue engineering, each modality has advantages and disadvantages that researchers must consider when choosing the best imaging technique for their research [77].

3.6 Photoacoustic Imaging

The shortcomings of conventional medical imaging modalities are being addressed by emerging imaging technologies, with photoacoustic (PA) imaging showing particular promise. By transforming optical energy into ultrasonic energy, PA imaging combines the benefits of both optical and ultrasonic imaging in a unique way. In this procedure, biological tissues are exposed to nanosecond laser pulses, which cause thermoelastic expansion and a brief rise in temperature. This results in the production of acoustic waves, which may be picked up by piezoelectric sensors or ultrasonic transducers. Because ultrasonic scattering is around three orders of magnitude lower than optical scattering, PA imaging has the potential to penetrate deeper, which is one of its major advantages. Unlike traditional optical microscopy, PA imaging allows for capturing deeper tissue features. Figure 3.5 shows the macroscopic and mesoscopic photoacoustic imaging techniques to monitor disease progression and vascular changes caused by treatment [78, 79]. In patient-derived xenografts of head and neck (H&N) cancer, tumor oxygen saturation (sO_2) was identified as an early marker of response to EBRT, with higher sO_2 levels indicating a positive response to single-dose radiation treatment [78, 79]. Furthermore, PA imaging extends its use beyond subcellular to whole-animal investigations by allowing researchers to manage the trade-off between penetration depth and spatial resolution. In contrast to conventional ultrasound imaging, PA imaging provides a range of choices for both endogenous and exogenous contrast agents, including as metallic nanoparticles, melanin, hemoglobin, and other colors. Applications like as blood vessel imaging and the monitoring of tagged cells and proteins are made easier by this flexibility, which makes it possible to get functional and molecular information [79, 80]. PA microscopy is a useful technique for the nondestructive evaluation of tissue-engineered objects in vitro since it operates at subcellular spatial resolutions with comparatively shallow penetration depths (less than 1 mm).

For example, research has demonstrated that single-walled carbon nanotube-containing tissue-engineered polymer scaffolds perform better than micro-CT in terms of quantitative scaffold analysis and imaging contrast. Using dyes, gold nanoparticles, or the potent endogenous optical absorption of melanoma cells, PA imaging has also been utilized to observe the spatial distribution of various cell types over time within manmade structures. Several technologies, such as linear array-based imaging, tomographic techniques, and single-element transducer-based microscopy, have shown the value of PA imaging in vivo. As demonstrated in models such as the naked mouse ear, PA microscopy's great spatial resolution and sensitivity allow it to monitor vascularization and scaffold deterioration efficiently. Furthermore, bigger animal models, such as rats frequently employed in tissue regeneration investigations, can benefit from linear ultrasonic array-based PA imaging since it can identify targets at deeper depths [81].

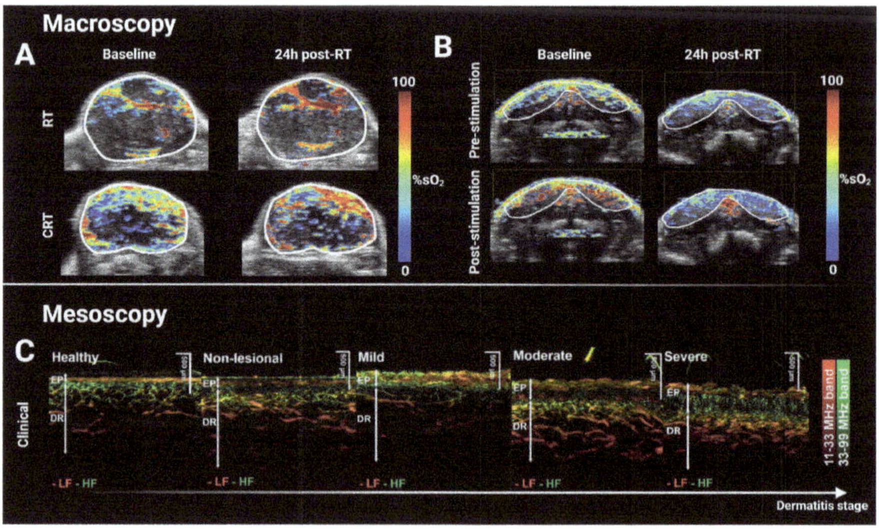

Fig. 3.5 **a** A quantitative blood oxygen saturation (sO_2) map, derived from multispectral optoacoustic tomography (MSOT). **b** A salivary gland hemodynamic stimulation challenge, conducted before and after a single 15 Gy dose, showed a diminished sO_2 response after radiation therapy, indicating radiation-induced damage. **c** Mesoscopic photoacoustic imaging (PAI) of graded atopic dermatitis in human skin, visualized by a clinical XZ maximum intensity projection, demonstrated how vascular and structural scoring could be used to grade dermatitis and assess radiation-induced toxicity in radiotherapy (RT). Figure reproduced under license CC-BY-4.0 [79] (https://creativecommons.org/licenses/by/4.0/)

The delivery of mesenchymal stem cells tagged with gold nanospheres to ischemic muscle tissues in PEGylated fibrin gel for long-term monitoring is a noteworthy example. This application demonstrates how PA imaging may be used to monitor cellular interactions and behavior over time in vivo. Photoacoustic imaging is a breakthrough in biomedical imaging, providing researchers in tissue engineering and regenerative medicine with a flexible and potent tool that advances the knowledge of biological processes and treatment approaches [82].

3.7 Multimodal Imaging

The limitations of individual imaging modalities are being effectively addressed by multimodal imaging methodologies, especially when studying tissue-engineered constructions. Every imaging approach has limitations, and no single technique can fully offer all the needed information. Researchers can acquire a more comprehensive image involving morphological, functional, and molecular data by integrating several imaging modalities [83]. Many imaging modalities, including CT/PET, CT/SPECT, MRI/CT, MRI/PET, MRI/fluorescence, ultrasound/photoacoustic (PA), and PA/OCT, have been integrated due to recent developments. To improve the visibility of artificial tissue constructions, several combinations are being investigated for preclinical and clinical applications. The creation of several multimodal contrast agents has further enabled these developments, which are crucial for effectively integrating imaging systems [84]. CT/nuclear medicine is one of the most often used multimodal imaging techniques in clinical settings. Because of their similar components, techniques such as PET/CT and SPECT/CT may be coupled efficiently to provide structural insights from CT and vital functional information about cellular and tissue activity. One research study, for instance, used PET/CT to track changes in bone formation and matrix metalloproteinase levels over time after BMP-induced cell injections. Similarly, utilizing SPECT/CT, the migration of human mesenchymal stem cells tagged with 111In-oxine was monitored in vivo for 48 h following implantation in rat tibia [85]. Furthermore, MRI has been used with other modalities like optical imaging, PET, and X-rays. Researchers are investigating multimodal contrast agents based on magnetic materials. While radiolabeling superparamagnetic iron oxide nanoparticles (SPION) with ^{64}Cu enables in vivo MRI/PET imaging, gold nanoparticles complexed with gadolinium function as dual contrast agents for MRI and X-ray. This combination of PET and MRI addresses the limited spatial resolution of PET and the low sensitivity of MRI. Additionally, much research is being done on dual MRI/optical imaging using iron oxide nanoparticles in conjunction with fluorescence or luminescence imaging agents.

Because PA imaging and ultrasound imaging share identical transducer and data-collecting methods, PA imaging also has great potential for multimodal applications. This combination enables non-invasive monitoring of implanted tissue-engineered constructions by combining structural data from ultrasound with functional and molecular data from photoacoustic imaging. Dual contrast agents for combined PA and ultrasound imaging, such as indocyanine green loaded into perfluorocarbon nanodroplets, are recent inventions. Furthermore, structural information can be improved by integrating hybrid PA imaging with other optical modalities, such as OCT. In conclusion, multimodal imaging, which combines several methods and contrast agents to enhance the viewing and evaluation of tissue-engineered constructions, is a promising development in biomedical imaging.

3.8 Conclusions

Advanced biomedical imaging technologies are essential to assess tissue-engineered constructions and regenerative medicine tools. These imaging techniques offer crucial details on regenerating tissues and tissue-engineered scaffolds, such as morphological alterations, functional information, integration with native tissues, growth factor release, and cell incorporation inside scaffolds. From subcellular to whole-animal investigations, this data is useful at many different spatial scales and has a wide range of applications, such as in vitro research and clinical situations. However, no one imaging modality can fully supply all the information that is required. Nuclear medicine and optical imaging methods, for instance, provide great sensitivity and functional insights, but they lack anatomical features and may have limits in imaging depth or safety problems. On the other hand, radiography and ultrasound imaging are excellent at giving detailed and high-resolution anatomical information, but they struggle with the efficacy of molecular imaging agents in various tissues. Although MRI helps with problems with contrast and penetration depth, its use may be hampered by its low sensitivity, limited selection of molecular probes, and high cost. Although not all needed data can be acquired by a single approach, researchers frequently have to select an imaging modality depending on particular informational demands and applications. By combining the advantages of several imaging methods, multimodal imaging offers a viable remedy for these constraints. Researchers may evaluate tissue-engineered constructions more thoroughly by integrating the best aspects of many modalities. Furthermore, the integration of biomedical imaging with tissue engineering has been further helped by developments in contrast agents that improve imaging contrast while also giving functional information. In conclusion, developing tissue engineering techniques and their therapeutic applications largely depends on sophisticated imaging technology. Researchers can greatly advance their knowledge of tissue-engineered constructions and their therapeutic potential by overcoming the drawbacks of individual imaging modalities using multimodal techniques and cutting-edge contrast agents.

References

1. Place ES, Evans ND, Stevens MM (2009) Complexity in biomaterials for tissue engineering. Nat Mater 8(6):457–470
2. Dvir T, Timko BP, Kohane DS, Langer R (2010) Nanotechnological strategies for engineering complex tissues. Nat Nanotechnol 6(1):13–22
3. Singh G, Chanda A (2024) Biofidelic gallbladder tissue surrogates. Adv Mater Process Technol. https://doi.org/10.1080/2374068X.2023.2198835
4. Singh G, Chanda A (2024) Development and biomechanical testing of artificial surrogates for vaginal tissue. Adv Mater Process Technol. https://doi.org/10.1080/2374068X.2023.2198837
5. Guagliardi A et al (2009) Toward the X-ray microdiffraction imaging of bone and tissue-engineered bone. Tissue Eng Part B Rev 15:423–442
6. Brenner DJ, Hall EJ (2007) Computed tomography—an increasing source of radiation exposure. N Engl J Med 357:2277–2284
7. Majumdar P, Singh G, Chanda A (2024) Development and biomechanical testing of full-scale human brain simulant. J Eng Res. https://doi.org/10.1016/J.JER.2024.02.016
8. Singh G, Chanda A (2022) Biomechanical modeling of progressive wound healing: a computational study. Biomed Eng Adv 4:100055
9. Jones AC et al (2004) Analysis of 3D bone ingrowth into polymer scaffolds via micro-computed tomography imaging. Biomaterials 25:4947–4954
10. Meinel L et al (2004) Bone tissue engineering using human mesenchymal stem cells: effects of scaffold material and medium flow. Ann Biomed Eng 32:112–122
11. Chanda A, Ruchti T, Unnikrishnan V (2018) Computational modeling of wound suture: a review. IEEE Rev Biomed Eng 11:165–176
12. Afazal M, Gupta S, Tevatia A, Afreen S, Chanda A (2023) Computational fluid dynamics-based model for assessing rupture risk in cerebral arteries with varying aneurysm sizes. Computation 11:79
13. Serafim A, Cecoltan S, Olăreț E, Dragusin DM, Vasile E, Popescu V et al (2020) Bioinspired hydrogel coating based on methacryloyl gelatin bioactivates polypropylene meshes for abdominal wall repair. Polymers 12(8):1677
14. Afazal M, Afreen S, Chanda A (2023) Computational modelling and analysis of hard tissue behavior around 0.5 mm and 0.85 mm platform switched abutment using 3D finite element analysis. Forces Mech 13:100243
15. Singla R, Gupta S, Chanda A (2023) A computational fluid dynamics-based model for assessing rupture risk in cerebral arteries with varying aneurysm sizes. Math Comput Appl 28:90
16. Ellahi A, Gupta S, Bose D, Chanda A (2025) A high-fidelity biomechanical modeling framework for injury prediction during frontal car crash. Comput Methods Biomech Biomed Eng 28:13–24
17. Bose D, Gupta S, Chanda A (2025) Scalable direct manufacturing of a functional multipurpose wrist-hand orthosis using 3D printing. Ann 3D Print Med 17:100186
18. Wang Y et al (2010) The synergistic effects of 3-D porous silk fibroin matrix scaffold properties and hydrodynamic environment in cartilage tissue regeneration. Biomaterials 31:4672–4681
19. Chhikara K, Gupta S, Chanda A (2022) Development of a novel foot orthosis for plantar pain reduction. Mater Today Proc 62:3532–3537
20. Chhikara K, Gupta S, Bose D, Kataria C, Chanda A (2023) Development and trial of a multipurpose customized orthosis for activities of daily living in patients with spinal cord injury. Prosthesis 5:467–479
21. Rothschild BM et al (2023) Design, manufacturing, and trial of a 3D printed customized finger splint for patients with rheumatoid arthritis. Rheumato 3:51–62
22. Giuliani A et al (2014) Polyglycolic acid-polylactic acid scaffold response to different progenitor cell in vitro cultures: a demonstrative and comparative X-ray synchrotron radiation phase-contrast microtomography study. Tissue Eng Part C Methods 20:308–316
23. Nath Yadav P, Singh G, Chanda A (2022) Biomechanical modeling of cerebral aneurysm. Mater Today Proc 62:3295–3300

24. Gupta V, Chanda A (2021) Expansion potential of skin grafts with novel I-shaped auxetic incisions. Biomed Phys Eng Express 8:015016
25. Yuan C et al (2024) Adipose-derived stem cell-based optimization strategies for musculoskeletal regeneration: recent advances and perspectives. Stem Cell Res Ther 15(1):1–24
26. Singh G, Gupta V, Chanda A (2022) Artificial skin with varying biomechanical properties. Mater Today Proc 62:3162–3166
27. Jiang C et al (2022) Biomechanics of skin grafts: effect of pattern size, spacing and orientation. Eng Res Express 4:015006
28. Gupta V, Singh G, Chanda A (2024) Modeling of metamaterial based incision patterns for generating high expansions in skin grafts. In: Lecture notes in mechanical engineering, pp 563–574. https://doi.org/10.1007/978-981-99-5919-8_51
29. Rahmim A, Zaidi H (2008) PET versus SPECT: strengths, limitations and challenges. Nucl Med Commun 29:193–207
30. Singh G, Chanda A (2024) Finite element modeling of diabetic foot: a state-of-the-art review. Eng Res Express 6:012507
31. Gupta V, Singh G, Chanda A (2023) Development of hierarchical auxetic skin graft simulants with high expansion potential. Biomed Eng Adv 5:100087
32. Almutairi A et al (2009) Biodegradable dendritic positron-emitting nanoprobes for the noninvasive imaging of angiogenesis. Proc Natl Acad Sci USA 106:685–690
33. Gupta V, Singla R, Chanda A (2023) Development and characterization of novel anisotropic skin graft simulants. Dermato 3:114–130
34. Gupta V, Chanda A (2023) Auxetic incisions with alternating slit shapes: a promising technique for enhancing synthetic skin grafts expansion. Mater Res Express 10:075802
35. Gupta V, Gupta S, Chanda A (2023) Development of an ultra-low-cost planar biaxial tester for soft tissue characterization. Biomed Phys Eng Express 9:025011
36. Zhou J et al (2010) The repair of large segmental bone defects in the rabbit with vascularized tissue engineered bone. Biomaterials 31:1171–1179
37. Gupta V, Singh G, Gupta S, Chanda A (2023) Expansion potential of auxetic prosthetic skin grafts: a review. Eng Res Express 5:022003
38. Gupta V, Chanda A (2023) Biomechanical modelling of hierarchical metamaterials for skin grafting. In: Materials horizons: from nature to nanomaterials (part F1471), pp 71–83
39. Gupta V, Singh G, Chanda A (2023) Modeling of metamaterial based incision patterns for generating high expansions in skin grafts. Clin Biomech 110:106118
40. Jun YW, Lee JH, Cheon J (2008) Chemical design of nanoparticle probes for high-performance magnetic resonance imaging. Angew Chem Int Ed 47:5122–5135
41. Gupta V, Chanda A (2024) Mechanical characterization of alternating slit, I-shaped and rotating triangle based auxetic skin graft phantoms. Mech Adv Mater Struct. https://doi.org/10.1080/15376494.2023.2250782
42. Chanda A, Gupta V, Gupta S (2024) Development and mechanical testing of auxetic incisions on human cadaveric skin, pp 89–99. https://doi.org/10.1007/978-981-97-4383-4_7
43. Chanda A, Chatterjee S, Gupta V (2020) Soft composite based hyperelastic model for anisotropic tissue characterization. J Compos Mater 54:4525–4534
44. Terreno E, Castelli DD, Viale A, Aime S (2010) Challenges for molecular magnetic resonance imaging. Chem Rev 110:3019–3042
45. Chanda A, Upchurch W (2018) Biomechanical modeling of wounded skin. J Compos Sci 2:69
46. Chanda A, Unnikrishnan V, Flynn Z, Lackey K (2017) Experimental study on tissue phantoms to understand the effect of injury and suturing on human skin mechanical properties. Proc Inst Mech Eng Part H J Eng Med 231:80–91
47. Chanda A (2018) Biomechanical modeling of human skin tissue surrogates. Biomimetics 3:18
48. Chanda A, Flynn Z, Unnikrishnan V (2018) Biomechanical characterization of normal and prolapsed vaginal tissue surrogates. J Mech Med Biol 18:1750100
49. Xu H, Othman SF, Magin RL (2008) Monitoring tissue engineering using magnetic resonance imaging. J Biosci Bioeng 106:515–527

50. Verma S, Chanda A (2024) State-of-the-art of finite element modelling of the human spine to study the impact of vibrations: a review. Int J Comput Methods Eng Sci Mech 25:225–247
51. Verma S, Singh G, Chanda A (2024) Development of a computational framework for determination of detrimental vibrations on the human spine segments. Multiscale Sci Eng 6(1):48–56
52. Verma S, Singh G, Chanda A (2023) A novel finite element model for the study of harmful vibrations on the aging spine. Computation 11:93
53. Torio-Padron N, Paul D, Von Elverfeldt D, Stark GB, Huotari AM (2011) Resorption rate assessment of adipose tissue-engineered constructs by intravital magnetic resonance imaging. J Plast Reconstr Aesthet Surg 64:117–122
54. Chanda A, Callaway C (2018) Tissue anisotropy modeling using soft composite materials. Appl Bionics Biomech 2018:4838157
55. Chanda A, McClain S (2019) Mechanical modeling of healthy and diseased calcaneal fat pad surrogates. Biomimetics 4:1
56. Ribot EJ et al (2017) 3D anatomical and perfusion MRI for longitudinal evaluation of biomaterials for bone regeneration of femoral bone defect in rats. Sci Rep 7(1):1–11
57. Ramaswamy S et al (2009) Magnetic resonance imaging of chondrocytes labeled with superparamagnetic iron oxide nanoparticles in tissue-engineered cartilage. Tissue Eng Part A 15:3899–3910. https://home.liebertpub.com/tea
58. Li W, Hong L, Hu L, Magin RL (2010) Magnetization transfer imaging provides a quantitative measure of chondrogenic differentiation and tissue development. Tissue Eng Part C Methods 16:1407
59. Ntziachristos V (2010) Going deeper than microscopy: the optical imaging frontier in biology. Nat Methods 7(8):603–614
60. Chanda A, Gupta S (2025) Healthcare entrepreneurship and management. Routledge, Taylor & Francis Group
61. Gudur M et al (2012) Noninvasive, quantitative, spatiotemporal characterization of mineralization in three-dimensional collagen hydrogels using high-resolution spectral ultrasound imaging. Tissue Eng Part C Methods 18:935–946
62. Wiskin J, Malik B, Borup D, Pirshafiey N, Klock J (2020) Full wave 3D inverse scattering transmission ultrasound tomography in the presence of high contrast. Sci Rep 10(1):1–14
63. Deffieux T, Montaldo G, Tanter M, Fink M (2009) Shear wave spectroscopy for in vivo quantification of human soft tissues visco-elasticity. IEEE Trans Med Imaging 28:313–322
64. Garra BS (2007) Imaging and estimation of tissue elasticity by ultrasound. Ultrasound Q 23:255–268
65. Yu J et al (2013) Non-invasive characterization of polyurethane-based tissue constructs in a rat abdominal repair model using high frequency ultrasound elasticity imaging. Biomaterials 34:2701–2709
66. Kumar VA et al (2013) Acellular vascular grafts generated from collagen and elastin analogs. Acta Biomater 9:8067–8074
67. Luker GD, Luker KE (2008) Optical imaging: current applications and future directions. J Nucl Med 49:1–4
68. Shachar M, Tsur-Gang O, Dvir T, Leor J, Cohen S (2011) The effect of immobilized RGD peptide in alginate scaffolds on cardiac tissue engineering. Acta Biomater 7:152–162
69. Tour G, Wendel M, Tcacencu I (2013) Human fibroblast-derived extracellular matrix constructs for bone tissue engineering applications. J Biomed Mater Res A 101:2826–2837
70. Chalal M et al (2009) Imaging the structure of macroporous hydrogels by two-photon fluorescence microscopy. Macromolecules 42:2749–2755
71. Podoleanu AG (2005) Optical coherence tomography. Br J Radiol 78:976–988
72. Yoon S et al (2022) Recent advances in optical imaging through deep tissue: imaging probes and techniques. Biomater Res 26:1–27
73. Ward A, Quinn KP, Bellas E, Georgakoudi I, Kaplan DL (2013) Noninvasive metabolic imaging of engineered 3D human adipose tissue in a perfusion bioreactor. PLoS One 8:e55696

74. Cowles EA, Kovar JL, Curtis ET, Xu H, Othman SF (2013) Near-infrared optical imaging for monitoring the regeneration of osteogenic tissue-engineered constructs. BioResearch Open Access 2:186
75. Onuma Y et al (2010) Intracoronary optical coherence tomography and histology at 1 month and 2, 3, and 4 years after implantation of everolimus-eluting bioresorbable vascular scaffolds in a porcine coronary artery model: an attempt to decipher the human optical coherence tomography images in the ABSORB trial. Circulation 122:2288–2300
76. O'Neill K, Lyons SK, Gallagher WM, Curran KM, Byrne AT (2010) Bioluminescent imaging: a critical tool in pre-clinical oncology research. J Pathol 220:317–327
77. Emelianov SY, Li PC, O'Donnell M (2009) Photoacoustics for molecular imaging and therapy. Phys Today 62:34
78. Luke GP, Yeager D, Emelianov SY (2012) Biomedical applications of photoacoustic imaging with exogenous contrast agents. Ann Biomed Eng 40:422–437
79. Lefebvre TL et al (2022) The potential of photoacoustic imaging in radiation oncology. Front Oncol 12:803777
80. Suggs LJ, Ricles LM, Nam SY, Emelianov SY (2012) Nonlinear photoacoustic signal increase from endocytosis of gold nanoparticles. Opt Lett 37(22):4708–4710
81. Zhang YS et al (2014) Non-invasive and in situ characterization of the degradation of biomaterial scaffolds by volumetric photoacoustic microscopy. Angew Chem Int Ed 53:184–188
82. Kim J, Piao Y, Hyeon T (2009) Multifunctional nanostructured materials for multimodal imaging, and simultaneous imaging and therapy. Chem Soc Rev 38:372–390
83. Von Schulthess GK, Steinert HC, Hany TF (2006) Integrated PET/CT: current applications and future directions. Radiology 238:405–422
84. Torresmartinderosales R et al (2011) Synthesis of $^{64}Cu^{II}$–Bis(dithiocarbamatebisphosphonate) and its conjugation with superparamagnetic iron oxide nanoparticles: in vivo evaluation as dual-modality PET–MRI agent. Angew Chem Int Ed 50:5509–5513
85. Emelianov SY et al (2006) Synergy and applications of combined ultrasound, elasticity, and photoacoustic imaging. Proc IEEE Ultrason Symp 1:405–415

Chapter 4
Ceramics Based Artificial Tissues

4.1 Introduction

Synthetic bioceramics, utilizing principles and techniques from the life sciences and engineering, are integral to tissue engineering for replacing, repairing, restoring, and enhancing damaged tissues or organs. The human body comprises various tissues and organs with distinct functions, and hard tissues form the essential framework that enables mobility and movement. Skeletal muscles, which account for 40–50% of an adult's body mass, are susceptible to injuries caused by trauma, lacerations, strains, contusions, or complications from surgical procedures. As the body ages, tissues can sustain damage or experience functional decline, necessitating surgical intervention due to their limited self-healing capabilities. Traditional treatments involve replacing damaged tissue with autologous tissue sourced locally or from distant sites, but these methods are constrained by insufficient donor tissue and risks such as donor site morbidity. Engineered scaffolds designed to use a patient's own cells to pre-construct tissue for implantation present a promising alternative to autografts, enabling the regeneration of functional tissue in vitro. Hard tissue engineering scaffolds are developed with specific mechanical properties and structures to promote cell adhesion, growth, and differentiation, leading to the formation of functional tissue [1–3]. For certain hard tissue engineering applications, the mechanical strength, porosity, biocompatibility, bioresorbability, and non-toxicity of implant materials need improvement. Recent advancements have also focused on creating antibacterial or anti-infective biomaterials to maintain sterility and prevent infections in scaffolds or implants. These biomaterials reduce the risk of infection, especially in procedures involving open fractures or bone remodeling surgeries. Microbial infections in such cases can occur as bacteria adhere to the material surface through various mechanisms. Passive adsorption is one such method, where interactions between bacteria and the biomaterial surface facilitate adhesion [4, 5].

As bacteria adhere to the biomaterial surface, biofilm formation begins, with bacterial colonization occurring during the initial stages of adhesion, depending on

A. Chanda and D. Sharma, *Handbook of Artificial Tissues, Biofabrication and Bioprinting, Volume I*, Biomedical Materials for Multi-functional Applications,
https://doi.org/10.1007/978-981-92-1307-8_4

the specific pathogen. Contamination can occur in both dry and moist environments, often spreading to bodily tissues through liquid carriers such as physiological fluids or synthetic solutions. Multiple factors influence bacterial adherence to biomaterial surfaces in aqueous environments, highlighting the importance of optimizing material properties to prevent microbial infections [6–8].

Variables: The adhesion of various pathogens, including gram-positive and gram-negative bacteria, as well as different bacterial species, can significantly influence the surface of implants. Factors such as the bacterial strain type and shape directly impact interactions between bacteria and biomaterials. These interactions are further affected by the physicochemical properties of the biomaterial, including its degree of hydration, hydrophilicity or super-hydrophilicity, hydrophobicity or super-hydrophobicity, the presence of hydrophobic functional groups, and the availability of functional groups. Surface characteristics, such as implant roughness and porosity (whether micro- or nanoporous), enhance bacterial adhesion. External factors, including electrolyte concentration, pH, temperature, fluid flow rate, viscosity, or shear rate, can either increase or decrease the surface activity of the material. These interactions contribute to the formation of biofilm on the implant surface, which acts as a reservoir for bacteria, leading to persistent infections. Once biofilm formation begins, it becomes highly resistant to antimicrobial treatments, making it difficult to eliminate [9]. To counter this, ceramics and other porous biomaterials can be engineered to produce antibacterial implants that prevent biofilm formation. Therefore, implants should be designed to possess both anti-infective properties and osteoconductive capabilities to promote successful integration and reduce infection risks.

4.2 Bio-ceramics

Bioceramics are a distinctive category of biomaterials designed to replace, repair, enhance, or treat damaged or diseased hard tissues in the body. Beyond their applications in medicine, ceramics are also widely utilized in energy, electronics, and optics. Porcelain, the first bioceramic material, was introduced in the eighteenth century for dental crown treatments. By the nineteenth century, plaster of Paris was being used for dental applications. The twentieth century marked significant growth in the use of bioceramics in medicine, driven by technological advancements. These materials are valued for their exceptional mechanical strength, slow degradation rates, and biocompatibility. Other notable properties include high melting points, low thermal conductivity, and resistance to plastic deformation, making bioceramics a highly compatible and body-friendly choice [10–12].

Producing an effective porous scaffold requires specific methods and parameters. Bioceramics can take the form of composites (such as polyethylene-hydroxyapatite), bioactive glass or glass ceramics (e.g., A/W), or polycrystalline materials (like hydroxyapatite or alumina) [13–15]. Due to their superior mechanical properties, materials such as calcium phosphate (CaO), zirconium oxide (ZrO_2), aluminum

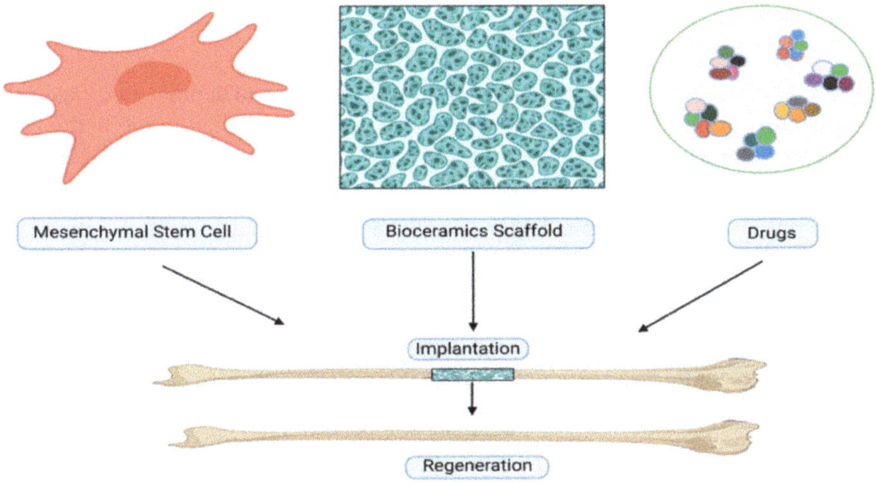

Fig. 4.1 A schematic depiction of the functionality of bioceramic scaffolds, mesenchymal stem cells, and drug delivery systems in bone repair. Figure reproduced under license CC BY 4.0 [20] (https://creativecommons.org/licenses/by/4.0/)

oxide (Al_2O_3), and bio-glass are widely used in the biomedical field, particularly in hard tissue engineering. Figure 4.1 illustrates a schematic representation of the functionality of bioceramic scaffolds employed in hard tissue engineering for bone repair. The bio-functionality and biocompatibility of these materials are vital to their effectiveness. Biocompatibility refers to a material's ability to elicit the desired biological response over the implant's lifespan. The success of an implant depends largely on the tissue's reaction to it and the material's behavior after implantation. The formation of apatite on the surface of bioceramics post-implantation enhances the bond between the implant and body tissue [16–19].

Bioceramics are categorized into three main subclasses: bioinert, bioactive, and bioresorbable ceramics [21]. Bioceramic materials are widely used in artificial implants due to their beneficial properties, although each type presents specific limitations. Alumina is commonly utilized in knee, hip, shoulder, elbow, and wrist implants for reconstructing fractured parts. It is valued for its high hardness and low friction properties, but its weakness in tension limits its broader mechanical performance. Zirconia is employed in hip and dental implants for similar reconstructive purposes. It offers advantages such as corrosion resistance, hardness, and reduced friction; however, it can suffer from friction-related issues and tends to be expensive. Bioglass is used in spinal fusion procedures to protect the spinal cord, but its brittleness makes it fragile under mechanical stress. Calcium phosphate and hydroxyapatite are applied in dental and bone repair as replacements for damaged teeth and bone. While they support biocompatibility and bone integration, they can also be prone to fragility under certain conditions [22, 23].

4.2.1 Bio-inert

These materials exhibit stable physicochemical properties and demonstrate excellent compatibility with hard tissues. In other words, when implanted in the body, they do not provoke a physiological reaction or trigger an immune response, ensuring they are not rejected by the surrounding tissues. They retain their physicochemical and biomechanical properties within the host environment, offering resistance to corrosion, abrasion, and fractures. Bioinert materials are primarily used as structural implants, such as bone plates and screws, to provide mechanical support. However, it is important to note that no material is entirely bioinert, as all substances elicit some level of response when implanted in the body. Alumina and zirconia have been widely used as traditional bioinert materials in dentistry and orthopedic applications since the 1960s [24–27].

4.2.2 Alumina (Al_2O_3)

The bioinert properties of alumina have been well-established since 1975. Alumina is known for its exceptional hardness and resistance to abrasion. Its crystalline structure makes it insoluble in standard chemical reagents at room temperature. Since the 1970s, alumina has been widely used in the production of artificial implants, notably in prosthetic femoral heads. The stability of alumina as an oxide is due to the strong ionic and covalent bonds between aluminum and oxygen. These bonds prevent galvanic reactions and corrosion, making alumina highly durable. Its excellent corrosion resistance, along with a low coefficient of wear and friction, can be attributed to its surface smoothness and energy. The hexagonal structure of Al_2O_3 is reinforced by aluminum ions occupying interstitial spaces [28–31]. The combination of abrasion resistance, strength, and chemical inertness makes alumina highly suitable for hard tissue engineering applications. Studies have shown no adverse effects on surrounding tissues when alumina is implanted in bone marrow. Enhancing tensile strength can be achieved by reducing particle size and increasing density. Synthesizing pure alumina has the potential to create a superior alternative to traditional surgical metal alloys. With its favorable mechanical properties, alumina implants contribute to extended longevity and durability in biomedical applications [32].

4.2.3 Zirconia (ZrO_2)

Zirconia was first discovered in 1789 by Martin Heinrich Klaproth and has long been used as a pigment in ceramics (see Fig. 4.2). It exists in three crystalline forms: monoclinic, tetragonal, and cubic. At room temperature, zirconia is found in its monoclinic form, while at elevated temperatures, it transitions to a tetragonal and then a cubic structure. The phase transformation from tetragonal to monoclinic enhances toughness, as the monoclinic phase is stable at lower temperatures. However, this phase change can compromise mechanical properties and lead to cracking. Partially stabilized zirconia, which retains sufficient mechanical strength, is suitable for medical applications, particularly in implant manufacturing [33]. Yttria-stabilized zirconia is a prime example, where yttria (Y_2O_3) is used to stabilize the tetragonal and cubic phases of zirconia, preventing undesirable phase transitions.

This stabilization enhances the static and fatigue strength of zirconia-based implant [35]. However, exposure to a single water molecule can trigger a phase shift from tetragonal to monoclinic, causing surface roughness and microcracking. Over time, this can lead to gradual degradation of zirconia femoral heads during implantation [36]. Nonmetallic compounds such as magnesium oxide (MgO), calcium oxide (CaO), and yttria (Y_2O_3) are often added to improve zirconia's stability. Zirconia's unique phase transition behavior enhances its toughness, making it highly advantageous compared to other ceramic materials. Its exceptional mechanical properties and wear resistance make it a preferred choice over alumina for certain applications. As

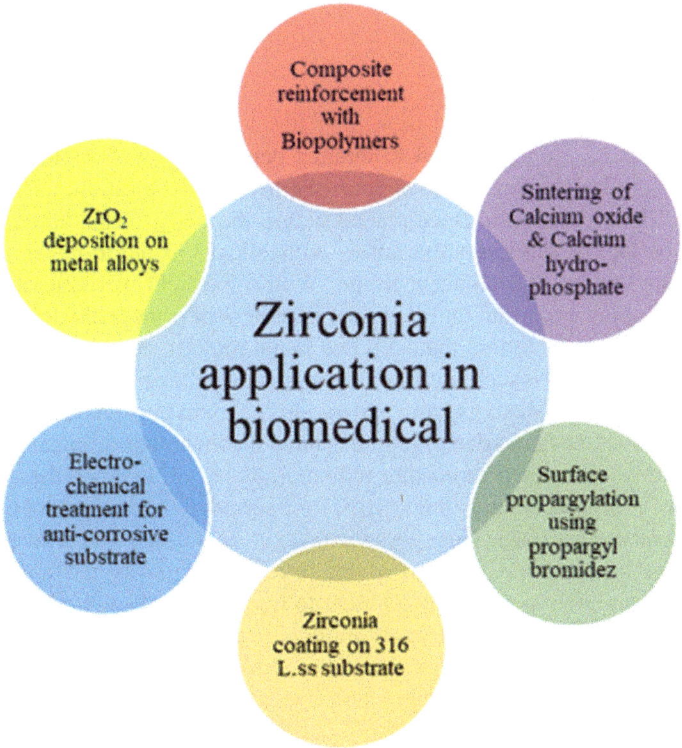

Fig. 4.2 Schematic of zirconia biomedical applications. Figure reproduced by under license CC BY 4.0 [34] (https://creativecommons.org/licenses/by/4.0/)

a brittle transition metal oxide, zirconia promotes early bone formation and integration. With favorable mechanical properties and excellent biocompatibility, zirconia has been researched as a biomaterial for the past 25 years. It is currently used in total hip replacement (THR), with ongoing advancements exploring its application in other medical devices [19, 37].

4.2.4 Zirconia-Alumina

Zirconia and alumina are notable for their fracture toughness and mechanical properties. However, water molecules can destabilize zirconia's surface grains, a process further aggravated by the presence of oxygen vacancies. To overcome the issues of surface instability and cracking, zirconia-alumina composites were developed [38]. These composites exhibit improved mechanical and morphological properties, with the addition of alumina playing a key role in stabilizing zirconia's monoclinic and tetragonal phases [39, 40].

4.3 Bioactive Materials

Bioactive materials are engineered to interact beneficially with biological tissues, stimulating cellular responses that support the healing, restoration, and rebuilding of damaged body structures. Once placed within the body, these materials trigger controlled biological processes that allow a chemical linkage to develop between the material's surface and adjacent tissue. Within the field of tissue engineering, such materials play an important role in the treatment of orthopedic defects, craniofacial bone damage (including the skull and facial region), dental applications, and persistent bone infections such as chronic osteomyelitis. Common examples of bioactive materials include hydroxyapatite and various calcium phosphate compounds. In recent years, bioglass-based dental implants have shown notable clinical success and are increasingly considered promising biomaterials [41, 42]. When these materials are immersed in simulated body fluid (SBF) for a period of time, a layer of hydroxylapatite forms on their surface. This synthetic layer closely mimics the mineral component of natural human bone. Because of this structural similarity, it can interact with collagen fibrils, allowing strong attachment to bone tissue. The interfacial reaction responsible for this bonding is strongly influenced by the chemical composition of the material, and even slight compositional modifications may significantly reduce or completely remove its bioactive behavior [43].

4.3.1 Bioactive Glass and Glass Ceramic

In 1969, Larry Hench coined the term "bioactive glass" and introduced its use. The primary components of glass ceramics are calcium oxide (CaO) and phosphorus pentoxide (P_2O_5) [44]. The presence of calcium (Ca) and phosphorus (P) enhances the bioactivity of bioglass, as they are essential constituents of the bone's mineral phase. Additional precursors, such as magnesium oxide (MgO), calcium fluoride (CaF_2), and sodium oxide (Na_2O) combined with potassium oxide (K_2O), have also been incorporated into bioactive glass with varying levels of bioactivity. To maintain bioactivity, small amounts of aluminum oxide (Al_2O_3) and boron oxide (B_2O_3) are sometimes included in the production process, potentially replacing silicon dioxide (SiO_2) [45]. Bioglass, a SiO_2–CaO–Na_2O–P_2O_5 system, is widely used in implant applications. It interacts with living cells, tissues, or organisms by chemically bonding to the skeletal system of the host. Upon contact with bodily fluids, bioglass forms an apatite layer, which indicates its compatibility with tissues and determines its bioactivity. This apatite layer promotes the formation of bone-like structures, demonstrating the osteoconductivity of bioceramic materials. The microstructure of bioglass also provides implants with high bending strength (215 MPa) and compressive strength (1080 MPa) [46, 47]. Figure 4.3 illustrates the unique application of bioactive glasses in the fabrication of multi-layered coverings that replicate the structure of cancellous bone. Bioglass compositions, such as 45S5, 58S, 70S30C, and S53P4, exhibit diverse properties due to their distinct formulations. The two primary crystalline phases of bioglass are silica and apatite. A calcium- and phosphorus-rich interface layer forms through a solid-state interaction between bioglass and bone tissues. This interfacial reaction, considered a chemical process, involves minor solubility of the glass ceramic material [48–50]. Additionally, certain glass, ceramic, and composite structures create a mechanically robust bond with bone.

4.4 Biodegradable Materials

These materials possess the capability to react and degrade rapidly when exposed to bodily fluids. Biodegradable substances are completely broken down by tissue fluids, which decompose their chemical structure. As a result, implants made from these materials do not require additional surgical procedures for removal. Once fully absorbed by the body's tissues, they become part of the hard tissue [52, 53]. The byproducts of ceramic resorption should ideally be processed through the body's natural metabolic pathways without causing any adverse effects. Numerous biodegradable implants composed of metals, polymers, and ceramics have been developed and evaluated in clinical applications. The controlled degradation of these materials offers significant advantages to patients [54–56].

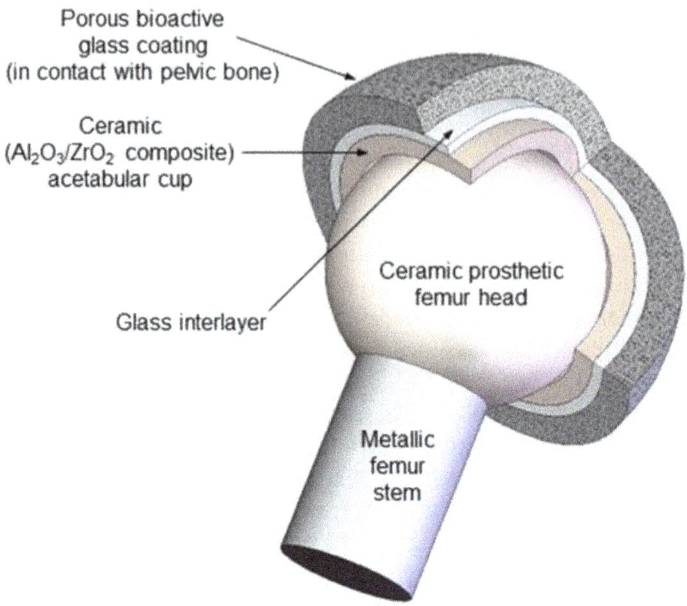

Fig. 4.3 The novel hip joint prosthesis features a single-piece, multi-layered acetabular component, wherein the ceramic cup is enveloped by a bone-like porous layer of bioactive glass, which may facilitate bonding with the host bone. Figure reproduced under license CC BY 4.0 [51] (https://creativecommons.org/licenses/by/4.0/)

4.4.1 Calcium Phosphate Ceramics (CPC)

Over the past two decades, calcium phosphate-based materials have been widely utilized in the biomedical field. These materials serve as the inorganic phase for bone minerals, aiding in the calcification process and the bone resorption mechanism, while exhibiting enhanced biological activity and affinity. For the last thirty years, calcium phosphate materials have been employed for bone tissue replacement in therapeutic applications, coatings, and implant fabrication. To be effective, calcium phosphate scaffolds must have a well-structured design with controlled porosity. Natural bone is composed of approximately 25% water, 60% inorganic mineral, and 15% organic mineral phases. Calcium phosphate can replicate the 70% inorganic mineral component found in bone [57–61]. The use of 3D planning significantly enhances scaffold manufacturing, resulting in scaffolds with improved mechanical and porosity characteristics that support cell adhesion and proliferation. In Fig. 4.4, the application of Calcium Phosphate Ceramics are shown where (a) hydrogel scaffolds integrated with whitlockite (WH), (b) cranial implants composed of tetracalcium phosphate and β-tricalcium phosphate (β-TCP), (c) injectable formulations containing calcium phosphate nanoparticles, (d) dental implants coated with a zirconia-calcium phosphate composite layer, (e) 3D-printed scaffolds made from calcium-deficient hydroxyapatite (HAP), and (f) 3D-printed structures using calcium

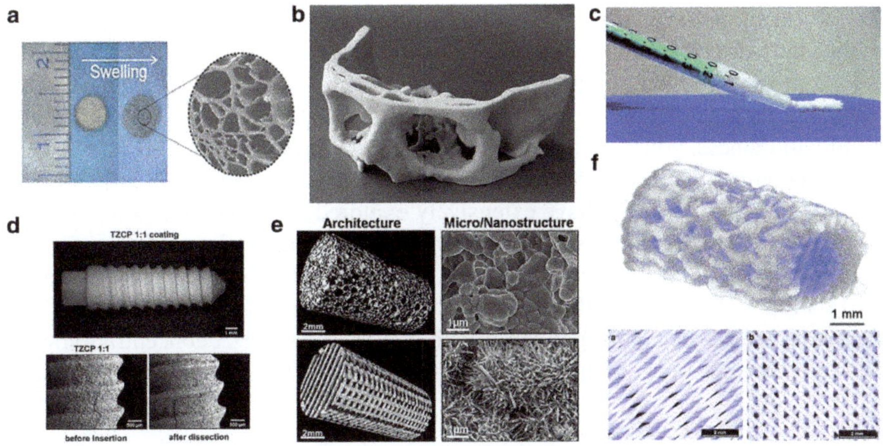

Fig. 4.4 Calcium phosphate-based technologies are applied in several biomedical applications. Figure reproduced by under license CC BY 4.0 [73] (https://creativecommons.org/licenses/by/4.0/)

phosphate cement. The microstructure and morphology of scaffolds and composites are analyzed using electron microscopy. Bone mineral crystals are small with a large surface area, but calcium phosphate biomaterials, in contrast, have strong crystal bonds and minimal surface area. The excellent stability, biocompatibility, and osteoconductivity of hydroxyapatite and β-tricalcium phosphate expand their applications in tissue regeneration. Composites and porous calcium phosphate act as carriers for biological agents, ions, and drugs, making them suitable for tissue engineering applications. Furthermore, the high porosity and biological properties of amorphous calcium phosphate and poly(lactic acid) nanofiber composites make them ideal for sustained ion release [62–66].

4.4.2 Hydroxyapatite

Synthetic hydroxyapatite ($Ca_{10}(PO_4)_6(OH)_2$) is commonly utilized in bone restoration due to its resemblance to the natural mineral apatite found in human bones. It is an alloplastic hexagonal material, crystalline in structure, and highly biocompatible, with a composition closely mirroring that of natural bone. Hydroxyapatite has a stoichiometric Ca/P atomic ratio of 1.67, aligning its chemistry with the mineralized phase of bone. It forms a strong bond with bone tissue by exhibiting an osteoconductive effect and excellent biocompatibility [67, 68]. Although hydroxyapatite shares significant compositional similarities with bone, its mechanical properties are inferior. Recent advancements have focused on hydroxyapatite powder as a means to improve its mechanical and biological characteristics at the nanoscale. Several techniques, such as hydrothermal synthesis [69], microemulsion [70], sol-gel methods

[71], co-precipitation, and mechanochemical processes [72], have been explored for producing hydroxyapatite particles in the nanometer range.

Hydroxyapatite also efficiently transports growth factors and osteogenic cells, enhancing its potential as a carrier. However, it has a lower Young's modulus and fracture toughness, which contribute to its inherently brittle nature [74]. The exceptional biocompatibility of hydroxyapatite (HA) is a key factor in its use as an implant material. Numerous studies have extensively explored and documented its biocompatibility. X-ray diffraction (XRD) analysis confirmed that the freeze-drying method produced HA without any contamination. Lee and colleagues successfully developed six types of crack-free HA scaffolds, demonstrating that the crystallinity of HA was preserved across all designs. Additionally, variations in HA concentration were found to influence the porosity of the scaffolds [9, 75–77].

4.5 Properties of Bio-ceramic Materials

4.5.1 Mechanical Properties

Each bioceramic material possesses distinct characteristics enabling a wide range of biomedical applications. The utility of these materials is determined by their biological compatibility and resistance to corrosion. Glass ceramics are particularly advantageous as they are biocompatible and easily bond with bone without causing harm. Consequently, the combination of inert and bioactive properties enhances the functionality of these materials. Additionally, these composites can exhibit improved mechanical and biological performance. Various biomaterials used in biomedical applications exhibit distinct physical and mechanical properties that influence their suitability for specific implants. Alumina has a density ranging from 3.3 to 3.9 g/cm^3, a high bond strength of 300–400 GPa, impressive compressive strength between 2000 and 5000 MPa, and a Young's modulus of 260–410 GPa, indicating its stiffness and strength. Zirconia is denser at 6.0 g/cm^3 and offers a bond strength of 200–500 GPa with a compressive strength of around 2000 MPa and a Young's modulus between 150 and 200 GPa, making it suitable for load-bearing applications. Bioglass, with a lower density of 2.5 g/cm^3, has a bond strength of 50 GPa, compressive strength of 600 MPa, and Young's modulus of 75 GPa, reflecting its brittleness and lower load-bearing capacity. Hydroxyapatite, closely resembling natural bone, has a density of 3.1 g/cm^3, bond strength of 120 GPa, compressive strength ranging from 500 to 1000 MPa, and a Young's modulus of 73–117 GPa. Glass ceramics offer balanced properties with a density of 2.8 g/cm^3, bond strength of 215 GPa, compressive strength of 1080 MPa, and Young's modulus of 118 GPa. In comparison, natural bone has a density of about 3.88 g/cm^3, bond strength between 60 and 160 GPa, compressive strength from 130 to 180 MPa, and a much lower Young's modulus of 3–30 GPa, highlighting the challenge of matching synthetic materials to the mechanical behavior of bone [78–80].

4.5.2 *Biological Properties*

(a) **Similarity with Bone**

Certain properties, such as composition, porosity, and mechanical characteristics, are designed to mimic the structure and functionality of bone in ceramic materials (see Fig. 4.5). The macroporous structure (100–500 nm) of bioceramics, along with their microstructure (1–10 μm), facilitates both tissue and blood vessel ingrowth during the formation of hard tissue. The interconnected pore network of hydroxyapatite derived from natural sources closely resembles that of bone. Conversely, synthetic bioceramics feature pores created using various techniques involving precursors. The final sintering temperature significantly influences the pore and crystal sizes in certain synthetic bioceramics. These materials degrade under cell-mediated acidic environments. The degradation behavior of both natural and synthetic bioceramics, whether in vitro or in vivo, depends on their structural composition, porosity, specific surface area, and crystallinity. Bioceramic scaffolds promote new bone formation through their osteoconductive and osteoinductive properties, enabling bone cell migration, adhesion, and proliferation. Bioceramic scaffolds exhibit mechanical properties comparable to natural bone. However, scaffold composition and particle size influence their performance and can impede hard tissue development [12, 81–83].

(b) **Bioactivity**

Different materials exhibit varying degrees of bioactivity, defined as their capacity to interact and bond with living tissues, which in turn can lead to different immune responses within the body. This bioactive behavior is largely determined by the material's physicochemical characteristics and surface morphology. Bioceramics, an important class of inorganic materials that may originate from biological sources or be synthetically produced, are widely recognized as effective substitutes for traditional bone grafts such as autografts and allografts. Notable examples include bioactive glass and several calcium phosphate-based ceramics, both of which show strong potential for biomedical applications. The composition and manufacturing techniques used to produce bioceramics play a crucial role in determining their biological performance and degree of bioactivity [85].

When bioceramics are placed in physiological environments, they gradually release calcium and phosphate ions that contribute to the formation of a calcium–phosphate (Ca–P) layer on the material surface. During this dissolution process, additional ions such as magnesium (Mg^{2+}), potassium (K^{+}), carbonate (CO_3^{2-}), and chloride (Cl^{-}) may also become incorporated, leading to the development of calcium phosphate crystals that support bone mineralization and deposition. Analytical techniques such as scanning electron microscopy (SEM) combined with energy-dispersive X-ray spectroscopy (EDX) have confirmed the formation of these Ca/P layers, which play an important role in enhancing cellular attachment to the biomaterial surface [8, 86–88].

Bioceramics interact with surrounding tissues through several distinct mechanisms of attachment. First, dense and chemically inert surfaces can support cell

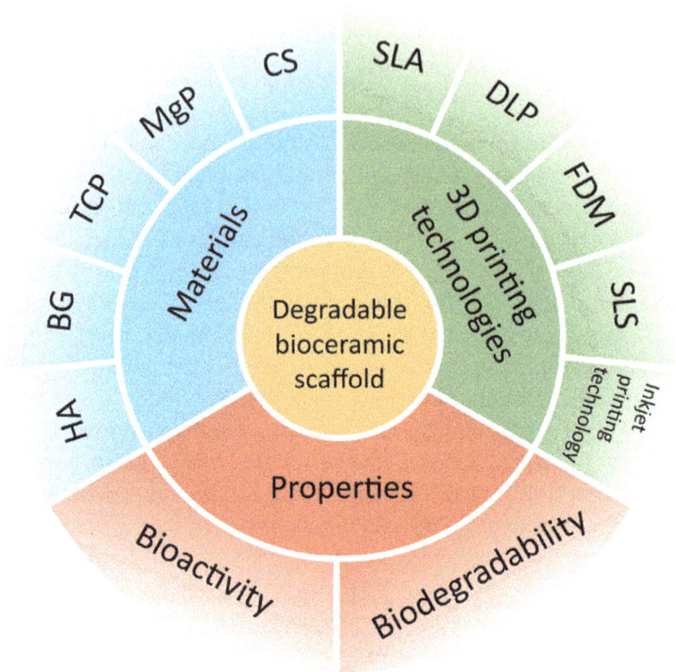

Fig. 4.5 Properties of bio-ceramic materials. Figure reproduced by under license CC BY 3.0 [84] (https://creativecommons.org/licenses/by/3.0/)

adhesion and tissue growth. Second, porous structures permit the infiltration and growth of new tissue within the material. Third, certain dense phases enable direct bonding to tissue through chemical interactions at the interface. Finally, some bioceramics gradually degrade, allowing them to integrate with and be replaced by natural tissue over time. The porous outer regions of the material improve mechanical interlocking with surrounding tissue, whereas the denser internal structure provides the necessary strength to bear mechanical loads.

The biological performance of these materials can be further improved by incorporating bioactive molecules or biological agents into the biomaterial system. Such additions can modify the surface chemistry of ceramic materials, increasing their biological functionality. Because the chemical composition of many bioceramics resembles the mineral phase of natural bone, bone-forming cells readily attach to their surfaces, promoting strong interfacial bonding. Studies by Hench and Andersson reported that the bonding strength between bone and certain bioceramics ranges from approximately 15 to 25 MPa, significantly greater than that observed with inert glass (around 0.5 MPa) or smooth titanium surfaces (approximately 2 MPa) [26]. As these materials slowly dissolve and release ions into surrounding body fluids, they can directly influence cellular activity and bone regeneration processes [89–91].

Cell attachment and spreading on scaffold materials can be examined using confocal laser scanning microscopy. Investigations involving hydroxyapatite scaffolds have demonstrated successful adhesion of pre-osteoblast cells, which subsequently develop bone-like structures on the scaffold surface. The observation of elongated filopodia and widely spread cytoplasm in these cells indicates strong cell–material interactions and highlights the excellent biocompatibility of hydroxyapatite-based scaffolds.

(c) **Biodegradation**

Cell-mediated degradation, also referred to as in-vivo breakdown, occurs in acidic environments and involves the activity of osteoclasts and phagocytic cells [92]. The degradation process is influenced by material properties such as composition, surface area, porosity, structure, and crystallinity. Additionally, it depends on factors like the pH, ion concentration, temperature, protein content, and buffer capacity of the physiological solution. The degradation of ceramic materials and the formation of an apatite layer on their surfaces have been studied using simulated body fluid (SBF), which mimics the pH and ionic composition of blood plasma due to its tris-buffer formulation. SBF is widely recognized as a reliable alternative to blood plasma for in-vitro testing. To assess the material's surface properties, chemical reactivity, and interaction with the solution, the material is immersed in SBF for a specified duration [93]. The formation of a hydroxyapatite layer in SBF confirms the material's chemical reactivity and functional ability to form bonds with host tissue cells. However, serum proteins such as albumin and globulins may inhibit the formation of the hydroxyapatite layer [86]. The development of a Ca/P surface apatite layer occurs through precipitation-dissolution processes, which can be analyzed using techniques like FTIR, SEM, and EDX. Biomaterials influence these dissolution-precipitation processes by altering surface charge chemistry, which can be measured using zeta potential after immersion in SBF. Once a calcium-phosphate layer forms, the material's surface charge transitions from negative to positive. By modifying these processes, the chemical reactivity, degradation rate, and mechanical strength of the material can be enhanced [94].

(d) **Bio Toxicity**

The development of advanced bioceramics has increased concerns about potential toxicity in the human body. Before bioceramics are used therapeutically, their effectiveness and biocompatibility must be thoroughly evaluated through cellular testing. Comprehensive mechanical, physiochemical, biological, and morphological studies are essential before material implantation to ensure implants have a long lifespan without causing localized or systemic toxicity. However, nanosized wear particles of bioceramics can sometimes behave unpredictably, leading to adverse effects such as osteolysis and inflammation over time. Consequently, toxicity testing of bioceramic materials is critical prior to clinical application [95]. Although testing bioceramic materials directly on humans would provide the most accurate toxicity assessment, ethical and legal concerns make this approach challenging. Prolonged contact between bioceramic implants and bodily tissues raises the risk of toxicity, necessitating a thorough evaluation of cytotoxicity, histotoxicity, and genotoxicity, particularly for permanent tissue replacements that directly impact surrounding tissues. To assess the biocompatibility of advanced materials, the FDA (Food and Drug Administration) and ISO (International Organization for Standardization) have established various methods, standards, guidelines, and procedures [96, 97].

According to ISO, verifying the biocompatibility of bioceramics involves three stages of clinical testing [98]. The first stage outlines protocols and techniques for assessing biological properties, including the selection of cell lines and mediums, extraction procedures, and controls. The second stage addresses animal welfare requirements for testing, while the third stage provides standards for test methods and associated challenges. While the FDA's testing criteria share similarities with ISO, there are notable differences in requirements and procedures. Non-clinical testing, including in-vitro and in-vivo studies of biomaterials, is conducted following GLP (Good Laboratory Practice) guidelines. Adhering to GLP standards is essential to prevent biocompatibility-related issues and ensure the validation of material biocompatibility [99].

4.6 Conclusions

This chapter provides an overview of both traditional and modern synthetic bioceramic materials used in hard tissue engineering. These materials enhance the compatibility, suitability, and durability of implants. However, further research is needed to improve the stability and performance of these materials for better patient outcomes. In particular, more work is required to enhance the mechanical properties of certain materials, such as bioactive glass ceramics and hydroxyapatite. Bio-glass and its derivatives are highly biocompatible and degrade rapidly within the body, but the mechanical properties of bio-glass-based materials remain a key concern. In some cases, metal-bio-glass composites may be used to provide the necessary mechanical strength. One of the main benefits of bio-glass is its ability to form an apatite layer upon contact with bodily fluids, promoting bone regeneration. Similarly, combining zirconia with alumina enhances both mechanical and biological properties, with alumina itself also offering strong mechanical performance. Hydroxyapatite is particularly beneficial due to its similarity to natural bone, making it ideal for both orthopedic and dental applications. While synthetic bio ceramic materials have both advantages and limitations, they are generally more advantageous than other materials. Bio ceramics based on nanostructures may hold greater potential for future applications.

References

1. Qazi TH, Mooney DJ, Pumberger M, Geißler S, Duda GN (2015) Biomaterials based strategies for skeletal muscle tissue engineering: existing technologies and future trends. Biomaterials 53:502–521
2. Kumar P, Dehiya BS, Sindhu A (2017) Comparative study of chitosan and chitosan–gelatin scaffold for tissue engineering. Int Nano Lett 7(4):285–290
3. Chanda A, Gupta S (2025) Healthcare entrepreneurship and management. Routledge, Taylor & Francis Group
4. Campoccia D et al (2009) The presence of both bone sialoprotein-binding protein gene and collagen adhesion gene as a typical virulence trait of the major epidemic cluster in isolates from orthopedic implant infections. Biomaterials 30:6621–6628
5. Chanda A, Flynn Z, Unnikrishnan V (2018) Biomechanical characterization of normal and prolapsed vaginal tissue surrogates. J Mech Med Biol 18:1750100
6. Arciola CR, Campoccia D, Speziale P, Montanaro L, Costerton JW (2012) Biofilm formation in *Staphylococcus* implant infections. A review of molecular mechanisms and implications for biofilm-resistant materials. Biomaterials 33:5967–5982
7. Merollini KMD, Zheng H, Graves N (2013) Most relevant strategies for preventing surgical site infection after total hip arthroplasty: guideline recommendations and expert opinion. Am J Infect Control 41:221–226
8. Chanda A (2018) Biomechanical modeling of human skin tissue surrogates. Biomimetics 3:18
9. Chanda A, Upchurch W (2018) Biomechanical modeling of wounded skin. J Compos Sci 2:69
10. Nath Yadav P, Singh G, Chanda A (2022) Biomechanical modeling of cerebral aneurysm. Mater Today Proc 62:3295–3300
11. Afazal M, Afreen S, Chanda A (2023) Computational modelling and analysis of hard tissue behavior around 0.5 mm and 0.85 mm platform switched abutment using 3D finite element analysis. Forces Mech 13:100243
12. Chanda A, Unnikrishnan V, Flynn Z, Lackey K (2017) Experimental study on tissue phantoms to understand the effect of injury and suturing on human skin mechanical properties. Proc Inst Mech Eng Part H J Eng Med 231:80–91
13. Davis JR (2003) Handbook of materials for medical devices
14. Turner IG (2009) Ceramics and glasses. In: Biomedical materials, pp 3–39. https://doi.org/10.1007/978-0-387-84872-3_1
15. Imran Z (2012) Bioactive glass: a material for the future. World J Dent 3:199–201
16. Luz GM, Mano JF (2011) Preparation and characterization of bioactive glass nanoparticles prepared by sol-gel for biomedical applications. Nanotechnology 22:494014
17. Gupta V, Chanda A (2024) Mechanical characterization of alternating slit, I-shaped and rotating triangle based auxetic skin graft phantoms. Mech Adv Mater Struct. https://doi.org/10.1080/15376494.2023.2250782
18. Chanda A, Gupta V, Gupta S (2024) Development and mechanical testing of auxetic incisions on human cadaveric skin, pp 89–99. https://doi.org/10.1007/978-981-97-4383-4_7
19. Gupta V, Chanda A (2023) Biomechanical modelling of hierarchical metamaterials for skin grafting. In: Materials horizons: from nature to nanomaterials (part F1471), pp 71–83
20. Tanvir MAH et al (2024) The role of bioceramics for bone regeneration: history, mechanisms, and future perspectives. Biomimetics 9:230
21. Kalita SJ, Bhardwaj A, Bhatt HA (2007) Nanocrystalline calcium phosphate ceramics in biomedical engineering. Mater Sci Eng C 27:441–449
22. Verma S, Chanda A (2024) State-of-the-art of finite element modelling of the human spine to study the impact of vibrations: a review. Int J Comput Methods Eng Sci Mech 25:225–247
23. Ellahi A, Gupta S, Bose D, Chanda A (2025) A high-fidelity biomechanical modeling framework for injury prediction during frontal car crash. Comput Methods Biomech Biomed Eng 28:13–24
24. Elsberg L, Moore M (1996) Total hip replacement: metal-on-metal systems. In: Clinical performance of skeletal prostheses, pp 57–70. https://doi.org/10.1007/978-94-011-0541-5_5

25. Hulbert SF (1993) The use of alumina and zirconia in surgical implants. In: An introduction to bioceramics, pp 25–40. https://doi.org/10.1142/9789814317351_0002
26. Hench LL, Wilson J (1993) An introduction to bioceramics, p 386
27. Chhikara K, Gupta S, Chanda A (2022) Development of a novel foot orthosis for plantar pain reduction. Mater Today Proc 62:3532–3537
28. Hong Z, Reis RL, Mano JF (2009) Preparation and in vitro characterization of novel bioactive glass ceramic nanoparticles. J Biomed Mater Res Part A 88:304–313
29. Singh G, Chanda A (2024) Development and biomechanical testing of artificial surrogates for vaginal tissue. Adv Mater Process Technol. https://doi.org/10.1080/2374068X.2023.2198837
30. Singh G, Yadav P, Chanda A (2024) Development of biofidelic skin simulants based on fresh cadaveric skin tests. Eur Burn J 5:454–463
31. Yadav P et al (2025) Gelatin multiwalled carbon nanotube composite 3D printed semi biological mesh for abdominal hernia treatment. Chem Asian J 20:e202401136
32. Al-Khateeb KAS, Mustafa AA, Faris A, Sutjipto A (2012) Use of porous alumina bioceramic to increase implant osseointegration to surrounding bone. Adv Mater Res 445:554–559
33. Piconi C, Maccauro G (1999) Zirconia as a ceramic biomaterial. Biomaterials 20:1–25
34. Nikkerdar N et al (2024) Recent progress in application of zirconium oxide in dentistry. J Med Pharm Chem Res 6:1042–1071
35. Nasser S, Campbell PA, Kilgus D, Kossovsky N, Amstutz HC (1990) Cementless total joint arthroplasty prostheses with titanium-alloy articular surfaces. A human retrieval analysis. Clin Orthop Relat Res 261:171–185
36. Chevalier J (2006) What future for zirconia as a biomaterial? Biomaterials 27:535–543
37. Gupta V, Singh G, Chanda A (2024) Modeling of metamaterial based incision patterns for generating high expansions in skin grafts. In: Lecture notes in mechanical engineering, pp 563–574. https://doi.org/10.1007/978-981-99-5919-8_51
38. De Aza AH, Chevalier J, Fantozzi G, Schehl M, Torrecillas R (2002) Crack growth resistance of alumina, zirconia and zirconia toughened alumina ceramics for joint prostheses. Biomaterials 23:937–945
39. Fabris S, Paxton AT, Finnis MW (2002) A stabilization mechanism of zirconia based on oxygen vacancies only. Acta Mater 50:5171–5178
40. Tsipas SA (2010) Effect of dopants on the phase stability of zirconia-based plasma sprayed thermal barrier coatings. J Eur Ceram Soc 30:61–72
41. Bhushan M et al (2015) Bioactive materials: a short review. J Orofac Res 5:138–141
42. Gheysen G, Ducheyne P, Hench LL, de Meester P (1983) Bioglass composites: a potential material for dental application. Biomaterials 4:81–84
43. Hench LL, Kokubo T (1998) Properties of bioactive glasses and glass-ceramics. In: Handbook of biomaterial properties, pp 355–363. https://doi.org/10.1007/978-1-4615-5801-9_22
44. Hench LL (2006) The story of bioglass. J Mater Sci Mater Med 17:967–978
45. Hench LL (1999) Bioactive glasses and glass-ceramics. Mater Sci Forum 293:37–64
46. Hench LL (1991) Bioceramics: from concept to clinic. J Am Ceram Soc 74:1487–1510
47. Apatite- and wollastonite-containing glass-ceramics for prosthetic application (PDF). https://www.researchgate.net/publication/32179241_Apatite-_and_Wollastonite-Containing_Glass-Ceramics_for_Prosthetic_Application
48. A review on recent applications of biomaterials (PDF). https://www.researchgate.net/publication/384054208_A_Review_on_Recent_Applications_of_Biomaterials
49. Jiang C et al (2022) Biomechanics of skin grafts: effect of pattern size, spacing and orientation. Eng Res Express 4:015006
50. Gupta V, Singh G, Chanda A (2023) Modeling of metamaterial based incision patterns for generating high expansions in skin grafts. Clin Biomech 110:106118
51. Baino F et al (2019) In vitro assessment of bioactive glass coatings on alumina/zirconia composite implants for potential use in prosthetic applications. Int J Mol Sci 20:722
52. Middleton JC, Tipton AJ (2000) Synthetic biodegradable polymers as orthopedic devices. Biomaterials 21:2335–2346

53. Wuisman PIJM, Smit TH (2005) Bioresorbable polymers: heading for a new generation of spinal cages. Eur Spine J 15:133
54. Ulery BD, Nair LS, Laurencin CT (2011) Biomedical applications of biodegradable polymers. J Polym Sci Part B Polym Phys 49:832–864
55. Singh G, Chanda A (2024) Finite element modeling of diabetic foot: a state-of-the-art review. Eng Res Express 6:012507
56. Gupta V, Singh G, Gupta S, Chanda A (2023) Expansion potential of auxetic prosthetic skin grafts: a review. Eng Res Express 5:022003
57. Kent JN et al (1982) Correction of alveolar ridge deficiencies with nonresorbable hydroxylapatite. J Am Dent Assoc 105:993–1001
58. Jarcho M (1981) Calcium phosphate ceramics as hard tissue prosthetics. Clin Orthop Relat Res 157:259–278
59. Verma S, Singh G, Chanda A (2023) A novel finite element model for the study of harmful vibrations on the aging spine. Computation 11:93
60. Gupta V, Chanda A (2023) Auxetic incisions with alternating slit shapes: a promising technique for enhancing synthetic skin grafts expansion. Mater Res Express 10:075802
61. Gupta V, Singh G, Chanda A (2023) Development of hierarchical auxetic skin graft simulants with high expansion potential. Biomed Eng Adv 5:100087
62. Guo X et al (2017) Porous Li-containing biphasic calcium phosphate scaffolds fabricated by three-dimensional plotting for bone repair. RSC Adv 7:34508–34516
63. Niu X et al (2017) Sustained delivery of calcium and orthophosphate ions from amorphous calcium phosphate and poly(L-lactic acid)-based electrospinning nanofibrous scaffold. Sci Rep 7(1):1–9
64. Chanda A, Chatterjee S, Gupta V (2020) Soft composite based hyperelastic model for anisotropic tissue characterization. J Compos Mater 54:4525–4534
65. Afazal M, Gupta S, Tevatia A, Afreen S, Chanda A (2023) Computational fluid dynamics-based model for assessing rupture risk in cerebral arteries with varying aneurysm sizes. Computation 11:79
66. Singh G, Gupta V, Chanda A (2022) Mechanical characterization of rotating triangle shaped auxetic skin graft simulants. Fac Univ Ser Mech Eng
67. Liu DM, Troczynski T, Tseng WJ (2001) Water-based sol-gel synthesis of hydroxyapatite: process development. Biomaterials 22:1721–1730
68. Bow JS, Liou SC, Chen SY (2004) Structural characterization of room-temperature synthesized nano-sized β-tricalcium phosphate. Biomaterials 25:3155–3161
69. Liu HS et al (1997) Hydroxyapatite synthesized by a simplified hydrothermal method. Ceram Int 23:19–25
70. Lim GK, Wang J, Ng SC, Chew CH, Gan LM (1997) Processing of hydroxyapatite via microemulsion and emulsion routes. Biomaterials 18:1433–1439
71. Horowitz SM, Purdon MA (1995) Mediator interactions in macrophage/particulate bone resorption. J Biomed Mater Res 29:477–484
72. Suchanek WL et al (2002) Mechanochemical-hydrothermal synthesis of carbonated apatite powders at room temperature. Biomaterials 23:699–710
73. Jeong J, Kim JH, Shim JH, Hwang NS, Heo CY (2019) Bioactive calcium phosphate materials and applications in bone regeneration. Biomater Res 23(1):1–11
74. Katti KS (2004) Biomaterials in total joint replacement. Colloids Surf B Biointerfaces 39:133–142
75. Lee H, Jang TS, Song J, Kim HE, Jung HD (2017) The production of porous hydroxyapatite scaffolds with graded porosity by sequential freeze-casting. Materials 10:367
76. Chanda A, Callaway C (2018) Tissue anisotropy modeling using soft composite materials. Appl Bionics Biomech 2018:4838157
77. Verma S, Singh G, Chanda A (2024) Development of a computational framework for determination of detrimental vibrations on the human spine segments. Multiscale Sci Eng 6(1):48–56

78. Singh G, Gupta V, Chanda A (2022) Artificial skin with varying biomechanical properties. Mater Today Proc 62:3162–3166
79. Rothschild BM et al (2023) Design, manufacturing, and trial of a 3D printed customized finger splint for patients with rheumatoid arthritis. Rheumato 3:51–62
80. Yadav P, Kamboj M, Das B (2024) Application of nanotechnology in antimicrobial coating on surgical instruments. In: Applications of nanotechnology in biomedical engineering, pp 150–168. https://doi.org/10.1201/9781003432661-9
81. Oonishi H et al (2000) Quantitative comparison of bone growth behavior in granules of Bioglass®, A-W glass-ceramic, and hydroxyapatite. J Biomed Mater Res 51:37–46
82. Livingston TL et al (2003) Mesenchymal stem cells combined with biphasic calcium phosphate ceramics promote bone regeneration. J Mater Sci Mater Med 14:211–218
83. Gupta V, Singh G, Chanda A, Chanda A (2021) Expansion potential of skin grafts with novel I-shaped auxetic incisions. Biomed Phys Eng Express 8:015016
84. Lin H et al (2023) Mechanism and application of 3D-printed degradable bioceramic scaffolds for bone repair. Biomater Sci 11:7034–7050
85. Alarake NZ, Frohberg P, Groth T, Pietzsch M (2017) Mechanical properties and biocompatibility of in situ enzymatically cross-linked gelatin hydrogels. Int J Artif Organs 40:159
86. El-Ghannam A, Ning CQ (2006) Effect of bioactive ceramic dissolution on the mechanism of bone mineralization and guided tissue growth in vitro. J Biomed Mater Res A 76:386–397
87. Bose D, Gupta S, Chanda A (2025) Scalable direct manufacturing of a functional multipurpose wrist-hand orthosis using 3D printing. Ann 3D Print Med 17:100186
88. Chanda A, McClain S (2019) Mechanical modeling of healthy and diseased calcaneal fat pad surrogates. Biomimetics 4:1
89. Pietak AM, Reid JW, Stott MJ, Sayer M (2007) Silicon substitution in the calcium phosphate bioceramics. Biomaterials 28:4023–4032
90. Ducheyne P, Qiu Q (1999) Bioactive ceramics: the effect of surface reactivity on bone formation and bone cell function. Biomaterials 20:2287–2303
91. Majumdar P, Singh G, Chanda A (2024) Development and biomechanical testing of full-scale human brain simulant. J Eng Res. https://doi.org/10.1016/J.JER.2024.02.016
92. Heymann D, Guicheux J, Rousselle AV (2001) Ultrastructural evidence in vitro of osteoclast-induced degradation of calcium phosphate ceramic by simultaneous resorption and phagocytosis mechanisms. Histol Histopathol 16:37–44
93. Kokubo T (1991) Bioactive glass ceramics: properties and applications. Biomaterials 12:155–163
94. Lu HH, Pollack SR, Ducheyne P (2000) Temporal zeta potential variations of 45S5 bioactive glass immersed in an electrolyte solution. J Biomed Mater Res 51:80–87
95. Thrivikraman G, Madras G, Basu B (2014) In vitro/in vivo assessment and mechanisms of toxicity of bioceramic materials and its wear particulates. RSC Adv 4:12763–12781
96. Sikalidis C (2011) Advances in ceramics—electric and magnetic ceramics, bioceramics, ceramics and environment. https://doi.org/10.5772/726
97. Anderson JM (2001) Biological responses to materials. Annu Rev Mater Sci 31:81–110
98. Murray PE, García Godoy C, García Godoy F (2007) How is the biocompatibility of dental biomaterials evaluated? Med Oral Patol Oral Cir Bucal 12:E258–E266
99. Helmus MN, Gibbons DF, Cebon D (2008) Biocompatibility: meeting a key functional requirement of next-generation medical devices. Toxicol Pathol 36:70–80

Chapter 5
Polymers Based Artificial Tissues

5.1 Introduction

From ancient myths such as Prometheus and Osiris to modern cinema like Pedro Almodóvar's *The Skin I Live In*, the concept of organ regeneration and bodily restoration has long inspired artistic imagination. In medicine, tissue engineering (TE) has emerged since the 1990s as a key interdisciplinary field aimed at repairing or replacing damaged tissues and organs, thereby advancing regenerative medicine. The fundamental goal of TE is to fabricate fully functional tissue constructs. This typically involves seeding living cells onto a scaffold that acts as a temporary substitute for the natural extracellular matrix (ECM), providing the necessary support for cell attachment, viability, and growth [1–3]. Scaffolds in TE can be fabricated from a range of materials, including metals, polymers, ceramics, or their combinations. The choice of scaffold material depends on the specific needs of the target tissue. Essential characteristics of TE scaffold materials include biocompatibility, biodegradability, appropriate mechanical strength, adjustable porosity, surface properties that support cell adhesion, proliferation, and differentiation, as well as sterilizability, nontoxicity, cost-effectiveness, and compatibility with minimally invasive procedures. Polymers, particularly synthetic biodegradable ones, have gained prominence in TE due to their mechanical versatility, tunable degradation profiles, high surface-to-volume ratios, and ability to be processed into a variety of forms. Synthetic polymers such as thermoplastics, elastomers, and foams exhibit a wide range of mechanical properties that can mimic those of native tissues. Because cells respond to their mechanical environment, matching these properties is essential for promoting tissue regeneration [4–6].

Compared to natural polymers, synthetic alternatives offer several benefits. These include adjustable mechanical properties, tunable chemical structures, compatibility with various fabrication techniques, reproducibility in manufacturing, affordability, and potential for delivering drugs or bioactive compounds. Conversely, natural polymers are often mechanically weak, non-thermoplastic, variable between production

A. Chanda and D. Sharma, *Handbook of Artificial Tissues, Biofabrication and Bioprinting, Volume I*, Biomedical Materials for Multi-functional Applications,
https://doi.org/10.1007/978-981-92-1307-8_5

batches, and difficult to purify, leading to higher costs and potential immunogenicity. Additionally, their degradation rates are harder to control due to structural complexity. However, synthetic polymers also have drawbacks, most notably the absence of inherent cell adhesion motifs. This issue is typically addressed by blending with natural polymers or chemically modifying the synthetic material to introduce biological cues. Many studies have investigated different polymer compositions to evaluate their suitability for TE applications, although systematic evaluations linking polymer type with regenerative outcomes remain limited. This chapter aims to bridge that gap by exploring the relationship between the physicochemical properties of synthetic polymers and their performance in tissue engineering. It gives the essential criteria for using synthetic polymers as scaffolds and discusses how these properties influence their functionality. Key synthetic polymers under study will be outlined, along with common scaffold fabrication methods. Furthermore, recent advances in preclinical applications tailored to specific tissues are examined, emphasizing the tissue-specific requirements for scaffold materials. Clinically relevant TE products using synthetic polymers are also highlighted. Finally, the chapter presents the perspectives on the future role of synthetic polymers in TE and offers guidance for researchers in selecting appropriate polymer scaffolds based on the latest findings [7–9].

5.2 Requirements of Synthetic Biodegradable Polymers

Biodegradable polymers, defined by their ability to degrade via biological mechanisms, are widely employed as scaffolds in tissue engineering (TE) applications aimed at tissue repair and regeneration. Among these, bioresorbable polymers are particularly valuable due to their complete degradation in vivo, which eliminates the risk of chronic inflammation [10]. Since the introduction of synthetic poly(glycolic acid) (PGA) sutures in 1971, various commercially available and lab-scale biodegradable polymers have been developed for TE use. The suitability of a polymer for a specific TE application depends heavily on the target tissue's mechanical demands and the scaffold's degradation rate, which should align with the pace of tissue regeneration. The chemical structure of polymers plays a crucial role in determining their surface characteristics, such as electrostatic behavior, wettability, and swelling ability, which in turn influence protein adsorption, cell interaction, and scaffold performance [11–13]. Initial cell-polymer interactions are mediated by protein adsorption on the scaffold surface, which affects cellular adhesion, migration, proliferation, and differentiation. Preventing nonspecific protein adsorption is vital, as it may provoke unwanted immune responses. The concept of biocompatibility has evolved over time. While early definitions focused on inertness, newer interpretations, such as that proposed by Crawford et al., emphasize a material's ability to guide cellular and protein responses toward functional, vascularized tissue integration without fibrotic encapsulation [14–16].

A scaffold's implantation initiates a host response that progresses from protein adsorption to inflammation and potentially fibrotic encapsulation, which can hinder vascularization and promote thrombosis. The duration and severity of chronic inflammation are pivotal—prolonged inflammation typically leads to fibrosis, whereas shorter inflammation can support tissue regeneration. Immunomodulatory biomaterials can mitigate fibrotic responses by regulating macrophage activity and promoting regeneration, a strategy referred to as in situ TE [17, 18]. Scaffold characteristics such as porosity and mechanical properties influence the immune response. For example, stiff porous scaffolds can promote anti-inflammatory macrophage behavior, while soft porous ones may induce prolonged inflammation [19]. Ultimately, biocompatibility reflects a spectrum of biological responses dictated by the physicochemical attributes of polymers, which are inherently linked to their molecular structure. Structural features like polar groups (–COOH, –OH, $-NH_2$) increase wettability and swelling, influencing degradation rates. Crystallinity, affected by polymer chain arrangement, enhances strength and stiffness but slows hydrolytic degradation, while amorphous, hydrophilic polymers degrade more rapidly. These relationships underscore the need for tissue-specific polymer design in TE applications [20–22].

5.3 Categories of Synthetic Polymers for Tissue Engineering

This section elaborates on the primary synthetic polymers used in tissue engineering (TE), focusing on thermoplastic polyesters, elastomers, and hydrogels. Each category includes specific examples with notable potential for therapeutic applications (see Fig. 5.1).

- ***Thermoplastic Polyesters***

Among thermoplastic polyesters, poly(ε-caprolactone) (PCL), poly(lactic acid) (PLA), and poly(glycolic-co-lactic acid) (PLGA) are the most widely studied and used in TE [23]. These polymers are typically synthesized through ring-opening polymerization of their respective cyclic monomers and are attractive for their FDA-approved biomedical applications, cost-effectiveness, biodegradability, and cytocompatibility [24–27]. PCL degrades slowly in vivo, over 2–3 years, due to its methylene-rich backbone, which may restrict its applicability in rapidly regenerating tissues. In contrast, the degradation of PLGA can be precisely tuned by altering the PLA/PGA ratio; for instance, a 50:50 blend degrades in 1–2 months, while an 85:15 blend takes 5–6 months. One concern with these materials is the acidic byproducts generated during hydrolysis, which can lower pH locally and potentially disrupt tissue regeneration, although this is mitigated in vivo by blood's buffering capacity. A major limitation of these polymers is their hydrophobicity, which negatively affects protein adsorption and cell adhesion. To improve their surface properties, strategies such as blending with natural polymers, like collagen, gelatin, elastin, or polysaccharides, and surface treatments (e.g., plasma modification or chemical grafting) are employed [28]. Additionally, copolymerization and blending approaches are used to

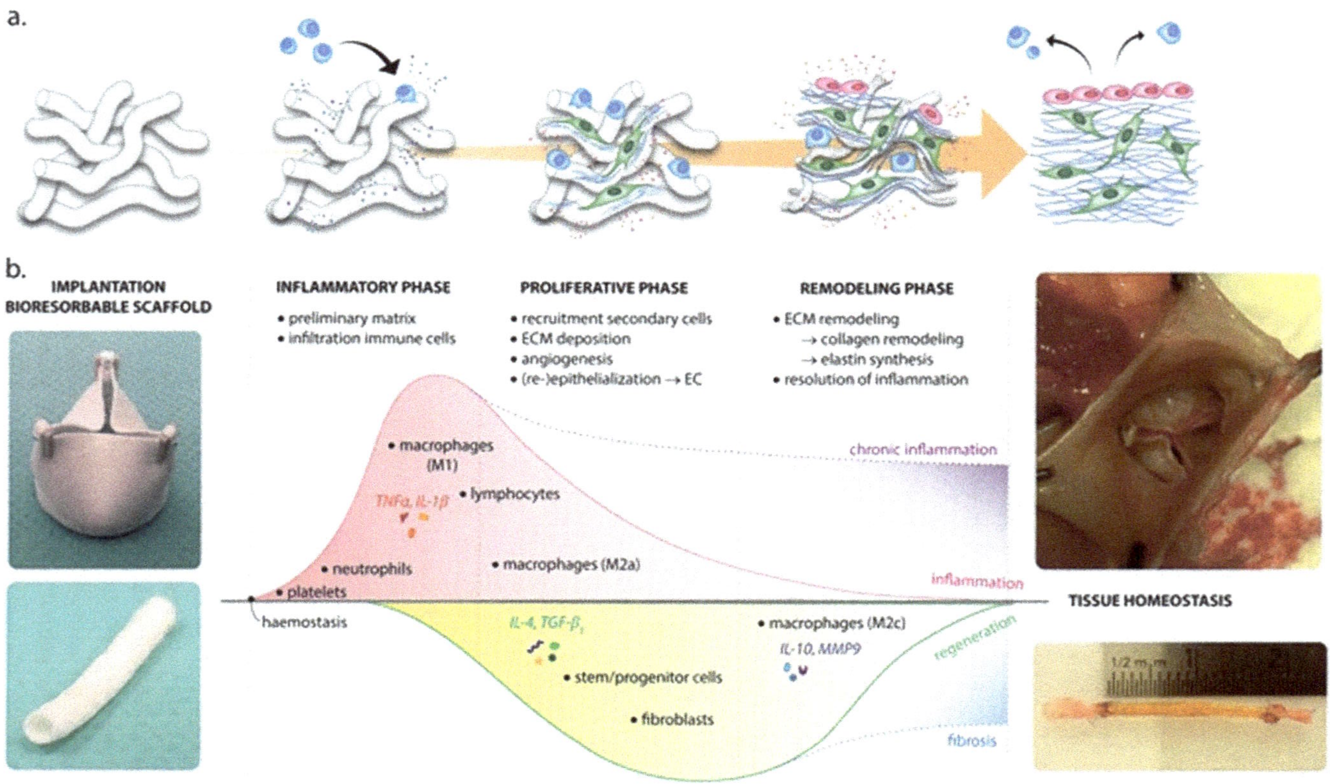

Fig. 5.1 In situ tissue regeneration mimics natural wound healing, starting with inflammation and immune cell infiltration, followed by tissue cell recruitment, ECM deposition, angiogenesis, and re-endothelialization. The final remodeling phase resolves inflammation and restores tissue homeostasis. Though not fully understood, this progression guides the design of regenerative biomaterials. Figure reproduced under license CC BY 4.0 [31] (https://creativecommons.org/licenses/by/4.0/)

tailor mechanical properties [29]. PCL and PLA have been extensively applied in scaffolds for bone, skin, cartilage, and cornea regeneration [30].

- ***Elastomers***

Elasticity is a vital mechanical feature for engineering dynamic soft tissues. However, designing biodegradable elastomers with adequate mechanical and biological performance remains challenging. Thermoplastic polyurethanes (TPUs), composed of alternating soft and hard segments, are promising candidates due to their tunable elasticity and mechanical properties based on segment ratios [32]. Typically, the soft segments incorporate PCL diols, enhancing flexibility and cytocompatibility [33, 34]. Recent advances include self-healing polyurethanes formed via dimethylglyoxime-urethane groups, synthesized without catalysts. Glycerol cross-linking modulates their stiffness to mimic various tissue types, making them suitable for in vivo applications like nerve repair and bone stabilization [35]. Poly(glycerol sebacate) (PGS), a polyester derived through thermal curing and polycondensation, is another notable elastomer due to its hydrophilicity and cytocompatibility. Modifying its hydroxyl groups with alkyl chains reduces its degradation rate. Poly(diol citrates), particularly poly(1,8-octanediol citrate) (POC), have also shown potential for TE applications [36]. Poly(trimethylene carbonate) (PTMC) is a rubber-like, amorphous polymer that degrades via surface erosion without acidic byproducts. Innovations like thiol-ene chemistry have enabled its application in 3D printing. Supramolecular polymers functionalized with moieties such as 2-ureido-4[1H]-pyrimidone (UPy) offer tunable mechanical properties and can be conjugated with bioactive agents through reversible hydrogen bonding [37].

- ***Hydrogels***

Hydrogels are hydrophilic, 3D cross-linked polymeric networks capable of absorbing large water volumes. Their swelling and mechanical properties depend on the degree of cross-linking: higher cross-linking increases strength but reduces flexibility and water uptake. Hydrogels based on poly(ethylene glycol) (PEG), poly(vinyl alcohol) (PVA), and polyacrylamides mimic extracellular matrix (ECM) characteristics, promoting cell proliferation. PEG is widely used due to its biocompatibility and stealth behavior. For hydrogel formation, PEG is functionalized with photopolymerizable groups (e.g., acrylates) or chemically cross-linkable moieties (e.g., norborene). Given its inert nature, PEG is often blended with bioactive molecules or peptides to enhance cell adhesion [38, 39]. Swelling behavior, essential for applications like vascularization, is optimized through tuning cross-linking density; excessive swelling can hinder endothelial network formation. PVA, derived from hydrolyzed poly(vinyl acetate), also forms hydrogels but has inherently low mechanical strength. Reinforcement with nanocellulose or incorporation of bioactive ceramics and natural polymers enhances its structural and biological performance. Synthetic poly(amino acids), particularly poly(glutamic acid), have been employed to form cryogels with large interconnected pores suitable for osteochondral TE. Ring-opening polymerization allows tuning of their mechanical properties by adjusting amino acid ratios [40, 41]. Composite systems combining poly(glutamic acid), lysine, bacterial cellulose, and alginate cross-linked with Ca^{2+} ions yielded a two-network hydrogel with cartilage-like compressive strength. Acrylates are seldom used in hydrogels, except for poly(2-hydroxyethyl methacrylate). However, poly(methyl methacrylate-co-methacrylic acid) demonstrated potential in chondrocyte culture and cartilage regeneration when combined with PEG-diacrylate and PEG porogens. This composite promoted chondrocyte phenotype maintenance and matrix secretion, offering promise for osteoarthritis treatment [42–45]. Synthetic polymers—including thermoplastic polyesters, elastomers, and hydrogels—offer tunable properties critical for tissue-specific scaffold design. Their chemical structures influence biodegradability, mechanical strength, and biocompatibility, which can be further optimized through blending, cross-linking, or functionalization to enhance TE outcomes.

5.4 Design Aspects, Polymer Selection, and Latest Advances

The design of a scaffold critically considers the chemical composition of the selected polymer, as it significantly influences its biocompatibility. As discussed in Sect. 5.2, a wide range of polymers has been studied for this purpose. The scaffold's morphology and surface properties also play an essential role in how it interacts with the surrounding tissues, making the selection of an ideal polymer particularly challenging. This complexity arises from the intricate nature of biological tissues, making it difficult to replicate their precise characteristics in synthetic constructs. Nonetheless, substantial progress has been made in understanding polymer–protein interactions, which has directly contributed to advancements in biocompatibility [46].

When developing scaffolds for tissue engineering (TE), it is essential to design architectures that physically and functionally replicate native tissues. In TE, scaffolds that incorporate constituents and microstructures resembling those of natural tissues have demonstrated superior performance in facilitating repair processes.

Chemical configurations of materials play a pivotal role in determining biological responses, and such characteristics have been extensively studied [15, 47–49]. Controlling these material attributes remains a well-established strategy for developing advanced biomaterials. For example, hydrophobic surfaces tend to absorb greater amounts of protein, often resulting in non-native structural conformation. Therefore, scaffolds with moderate wettability are generally preferred, as this preserves protein functionality and promotes optimal cell interactions. Additionally, surface charge influences scaffold performance—greater surface charge tends to reduce protein adsorption, which improves blood compatibility but may impair cell adhesion [50]. Since cell membranes typically carry a negative charge, positively charged scaffold surfaces can enhance cellular attachment. Mechanical properties, governed by the chemical structure's crystallinity and conformation, are equally crucial, as cells are sensitive to the mechanical stiffness of their substrate, which can influence gene expression. Moreover, specific chemical groups such as –OH, $–CH_3$, $–OSO_3H$, –COOH, and $–NH_2$ have been shown to produce distinct biological effects. Different tissues require unique scaffold properties, and the selection of scaffold materials must align with the functional demands of the target tissue. The following sections delve into the specific requirements of various TE applications and summarize recent findings in the field.

5.4.1 Synthetic Polymers for Soft Tissue Regeneration

Soft tissues such as cardiac muscle, aorta, and valves, along with connective tissues like ligaments, tendons, cartilage, and epithelial linings, each demand scaffolds tailored with specific mechanical and structural attributes [51].

- ***Adipose Tissue***

Adipose tissue, which can be either white or brown, displays unique mechanical characteristics based on its location and function. Due to the large deformations it experiences in vivo, scaffolds for adipose tissue must be both flexible and resilient. Effective scaffold design also requires interconnected pores greater than 100 μm to facilitate oxygen diffusion, angiogenesis, and nutrient transport. Among the studied polymers for adipose tissue regeneration are PLA, PCL, PTMC, and TPU. While PLA is mechanically strong, its brittleness limits its applicability. In contrast, TPU offers high elongation, excellent abrasion resistance, and a favorable Young's modulus. PTMC is particularly promising for adipose tissue due to its flexibility, low glass transition temperature, and amorphous structure. Copolymers such as P(CL-co-LA) and P(LA-co-TMC) enhance adipogenic differentiation more effectively than rigid alternatives like PLA and PLGA due to their greater elasticity. Novel elastomers derived from succinic acid, tailored by varying cis:trans double bond ratios, have also demonstrated enhanced degradation rates and flexibility, facilitating tissue regeneration. When compared to traditional PLLA, these elastomers promoted vascularization, cellular infiltration, and minimal inflammation after four months in vivo [52–55]. However, further comparisons are necessary with established polymers like P(CL-co-LA) and P(LA-co-TMC) to justify the higher synthesis complexity and cost.

- ***Muscle Tissue***

Skeletal muscle, which constitutes 40% of the body, has limited regenerative capacity. Scaffolds for muscle tissue engineering (TE) must encourage myoblast alignment, myogenic differentiation, vascularization, and nerve integration. Fibrillar scaffolds mimic native muscle architecture and support cell alignment and proliferation. These cell-free scaffolds are promising for in situ muscle regeneration due to lower cost and simplicity. Kim et al. demonstrated the utility of micropatterned PCL struts formed via PVA fibrillation in 3D printing to mimic native muscle microfibrils, supporting myoblast alignment and myotube formation [56]. Synthetic polymers used for muscle TE include PCL, PLGA, and conductive polymers like PANI, PPy, and PEDOT, which facilitate muscle contraction recovery and reduce fibrosis. To overcome processing limitations due to their rigidity and insolubility, conductive polymers are often blended with softer, more processable polymers like PCL. An alternative strategy involves incorporating conductive nanoparticles (e.g., gold or polydopamine) into injectable hydrogels formed from copolymers like Pluronic-CHO, which offer electroconductive, antioxidant, and antibacterial properties [57]. Despite their benefits, such nanomaterials may pose cytotoxic risks due to bioaccumulation, warranting their use only in highly specialized applications. An ideal scaffold for muscle TE should possess a Young's modulus of approximately 10 ± 4 kPa, mimicking muscle tissue elasticity [58]. Polymers like PEDOT-g-PCL are conductive, printable, and promote myotube development, making them excellent candidates. However, no perfect polymer currently exists, and further research is needed to develop materials combining biodegradability, processability, and conductivity.

- ***Blood Vessels***

Vascular scaffolds must support both large- and small-diameter vessels and reflect the structural complexity of native vessels, which include three distinct ECM-rich layers with elastic moduli ranging from 4 to 130 MPa. Electrospun nanofibrous scaffolds composed of polymers like PCL, PLA, PU, and P(LA-co-CL) mimic the native ECM and support endothelial cell attachment and elongation. Cell behavior differs with fiber diameter: smaller fibers (0.27–2.4 μm) facilitate robust adhesion and cytoskeletal organization, while larger fibers (> 4 μm) promote spindle morphology with reduced focal adhesions [59]. PCL remains a widely used polymer for vascular grafts due to its ductility and compatibility with suturing [60–63]. However, due to its slow degradation, it is often blended with faster-degrading polymers like PLGA or PGS. PGS, used as an inner layer in multilayered scaffolds, provides elasticity and encourages elastin production. Incorporating palmitic acid in PGS formulations has slowed degradation and improved graft performance in vivo. In tissue-engineered vascular grafts (TEVGs), host-driven immunoregeneration can eliminate the need for cell seeding. For example, PCL-PGS hybrid grafts have matched the performance of autologous vein grafts in rats. Additionally, antithrombogenic treatments, such as heparin or poly(1,8-octanediol citrate) (POC) coatings, enhance scaffold performance. Heart valve scaffolds are also advancing. Bioresorbable valves made from supramolecular thermoplastic elastomers like PC-BU retained functionality one year post-implantation in sheep [64]. These materials degrade slowly to match the extended regeneration timeline required for functional heart valve tissue, and their segmented structure imparts defined thermal and mechanical characteristics.

- ***Nervous Tissue***

The nervous system includes the central nervous system (CNS) and peripheral nervous system (PNS), composed of neurons and neuroglia [65]. While small peripheral nerve injuries (< 1 cm) can regenerate, larger lesions (> 10 mm) in both PNS and CNS show limited recovery due to inhibitory biological factors [66]. Synthetic nerve conduits are emerging as alternatives to autografts for peripheral and central nerve repair. These conduits must offer protection, support axonal regeneration, reduce scar formation, and enable high-quality regeneration [67]. Though FDA-approved synthetic conduits exist, their use is limited to injuries ≤ 3 cm. Notable examples include devices made from PLGA, PVA, PGA, and P(DLLA-co-CL) (e.g., Nerbridge, Neurolac).

Synthetic polymers allow tailored tuning of conduit properties, which should include biodegradability, flexibility, porosity, and conductivity. Soft, non-wettable surfaces support neural adhesion and differentiation, while conductive scaffolds must generate membrane voltage changes to trigger neurotransmitter release. Electroconductive polymers like PPy and PANI are valuable for enabling electrochemical stimulation of neurons [68]. Despite their potential, the clinical application of these polymers is tempered by challenges in processing and biocompatibility. Further innovations are necessary to improve neural scaffold safety, functionality, and integration. Synthetic polymer scaffolds for soft tissue engineering must be engineered with application-specific mechanical, chemical, and structural properties. For adipose and muscle tissues, elasticity and bioactivity are crucial; vascular applications demand compliance and hemocompatibility; and nerve conduits require conductivity, porosity, and flexibility. Although significant advancements have been made, ongoing research is necessary to develop synthetic polymers that can meet the complex demands of different soft tissues in clinical settings.

5.4.2 Synthetic Polymers for Skin Regeneration

Extensive research has been devoted to developing skin scaffolds that replicate the structural and mechanical properties of natural skin. Given the elastomeric and thin nature of human skin (1–4 mm), engineered scaffolds must exhibit high elasticity and durability to withstand surgical handling and suturing [69]. Key design parameters such as porosity, pore size, and wall thickness significantly influence cell behavior. Scaffolds with high porosity are beneficial for cell seeding and nutrient diffusion. The median pore diameter of a human acellular dermal matrix is approximately 95 μm, ranging from 96.8 to 131.2 μm, and pores exceeding 10 μm enable cellular migration within the scaffold [69–72]. An optimal skin scaffold should degrade within approximately 25 days to match the natural skin wound healing timeline [69]. Wettability is also crucial, as it supports scaffold–wound bed integration and promotes biological responses essential for skin regeneration [69]. Therefore, scaffolds should exhibit high hydrophilicity and water absorption capacity. Studies show that PCL combined with natural polymers such as collagen and gelatin, displaying low water contact angles ($\theta = 25$–$49.5°$) and swelling ratios up to 2000%, significantly enhances cell adhesion, proliferation, and differentiation [73]. In addition, skin scaffolds must retain their structural integrity and dimensional stability during clinical manipulation, while also providing a favorable surface for cell colonization (see Fig. 5.2).

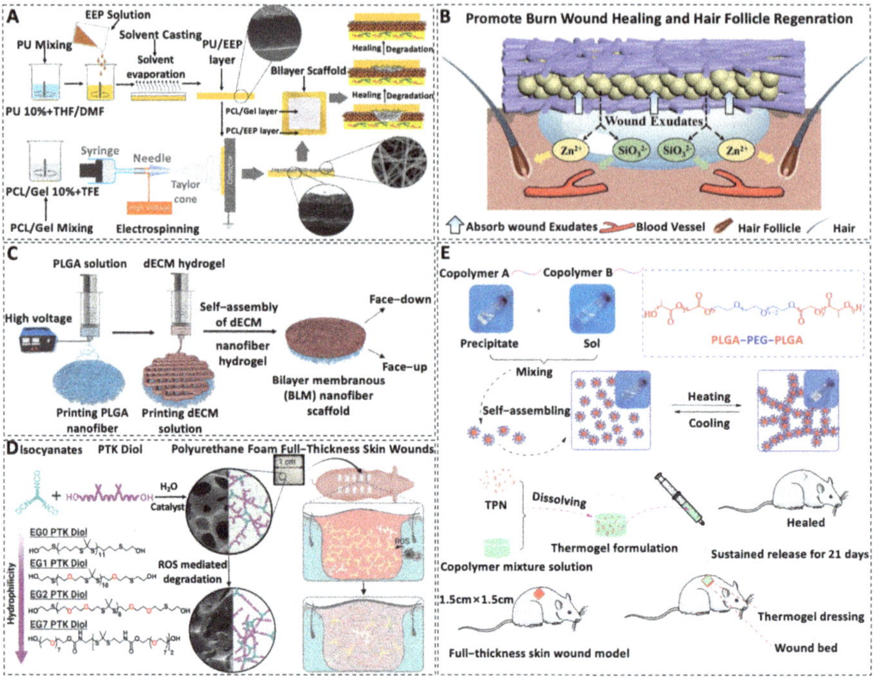

Fig. 5.2 Examples of polymeric scaffolds for skin tissue engineering include double-layer membranes using PU/EEP and electrospun PCL/gelatin, sandwich-structured dressings with zinc silicate and PLA, PLGA-dECM nanofiber composites to reduce scarring, PTK-UR foams with porous architecture, and thermogelling copolymer systems forming in situ hydrogels for wound healing and regeneration. Figure reproduced by under license CC BY 4.0 [74] (https://creativecommons.org/licenses/by/4.0/)

Synthetic polymers like PLGA, PLA, and PCL are extensively studied due to their favorable mechanical strength and ease of processing. Techniques used for scaffold fabrication include electrospinning, 3D printing, gas foaming, porogen leaching, phase separation, and fiber bonding. Among these, electrospinning is the most widely adopted for skin tissue engineering (TE). However, PLA's inherent hydrophobicity impedes effective cell adhesion and growth. PCL, noted for its chain flexibility and elasticity, is also widely used in dermal scaffold design, but its hydrophobic nature limits its ability to support skin regeneration. Electrospun PLGA fibers with diameters ranging from 350 to 1100 nm are most suitable for promoting fibroblast growth in synthetic polyester scaffolds [75–78].

While non-hydrogel-forming synthetic polymers provide structure and manufacturability, hydrophilic polymers like PVA and PVP are capable of forming hydrogels and incorporating active agents such as growth factors. PVA hydrogels demonstrate favorable fibroblast adhesion and possess skin-like mechanical properties. Both PVA and PVP are highly hydrophilic, allowing them to absorb wound exudates and resist environmental stress, which supports wound healing. Due to poor cell adhesion in many synthetic polymers, they are often combined with natural polymers, particularly collagen or gelatin, known for their regenerative properties even before TE emerged as a distinct field. Additionally, functionalized scaffolds such as PLLA electrospun mats incorporating europium and tannic acid have demonstrated enhanced angiogenesis, antioxidant activity, and improved hydrophilicity, leading to accelerated wound healing in rat models [79–82].

5.4.3 Synthetic Polymers for Bone and Cartilage Regeneration

Bone is a structurally and compositionally complex tissue characterized by gradients that must be replicated in tissue-engineered scaffolds for successful regeneration. Scaffolds designed for bone regeneration must satisfy several critical criteria, including mechanical stability, appropriate degradation rates, osteoconductivity, osteoinductivity, osteointegration, and antimicrobial capabilities (see Fig. 5.3). In terms of biomechanics, cortical bone exhibits a compressive modulus of 18–22 GPa, whereas trabecular bone ranges between 0.1 and 0.9 GPa [83]. While ceramics have been traditionally used for bone replacement due to their similarity to bone's extracellular matrix, their brittleness and lack of mechanical resilience have led to increased interest in polymer-based materials such as hydrogels, sponges, and meshes [83].

Scaffold surface hydrophilicity is crucial for bone tissue engineering (TE), as moderately hydrophilic surfaces with water contact angles between 55 and 75° enhance cell adhesion and osteoconductivity. However, synthetic polymers alone are typically insufficient to promote osteogenesis and are therefore often combined with natural polymers, bioactive ceramics (e.g., hydroxyapatite, tricalcium phosphate, bioglass), or growth factors. To enhance properties like mechanical strength and bioactivity, surface modifications and coatings are commonly employed. Additionally, copolymerization and polymer blending are strategies used to optimize scaffold attributes. ABA-type block copolymers—comprising stiff "A" blocks for mechanical integrity and flexible "B" blocks for increased hydrophilicity—are particularly suitable. Frequently used synthetic polymers in bone TE include PCL, PLGA, polyurethanes (PUs), PLGA-b-PEG-b-PLGA, and others such as polymethacrylates, poly(propylene fumarate), polyphosphazenes [84], and polyhydroxyalkanoates. The scaffold's 3D microstructure is vital during early osteointegration stages. While larger, interconnected pores (> 300 μm) enhance vascularization and cell adhesion, they may compromise mechanical integrity. Advanced fabrication techniques like electrospinning, lyophilization, 3D printing, and vacuum-assisted solvent casting are used to create such porous structures [85].

Research in bone TE is increasingly centered on composite scaffolds combining thermoplastic polymers with other components to capitalize on their synergistic benefits, and these composites are often 3D-printable [87]. Innovative cell-free strategies, such as decorating synthetic scaffolds with bone extracellular matrix using stem cells,

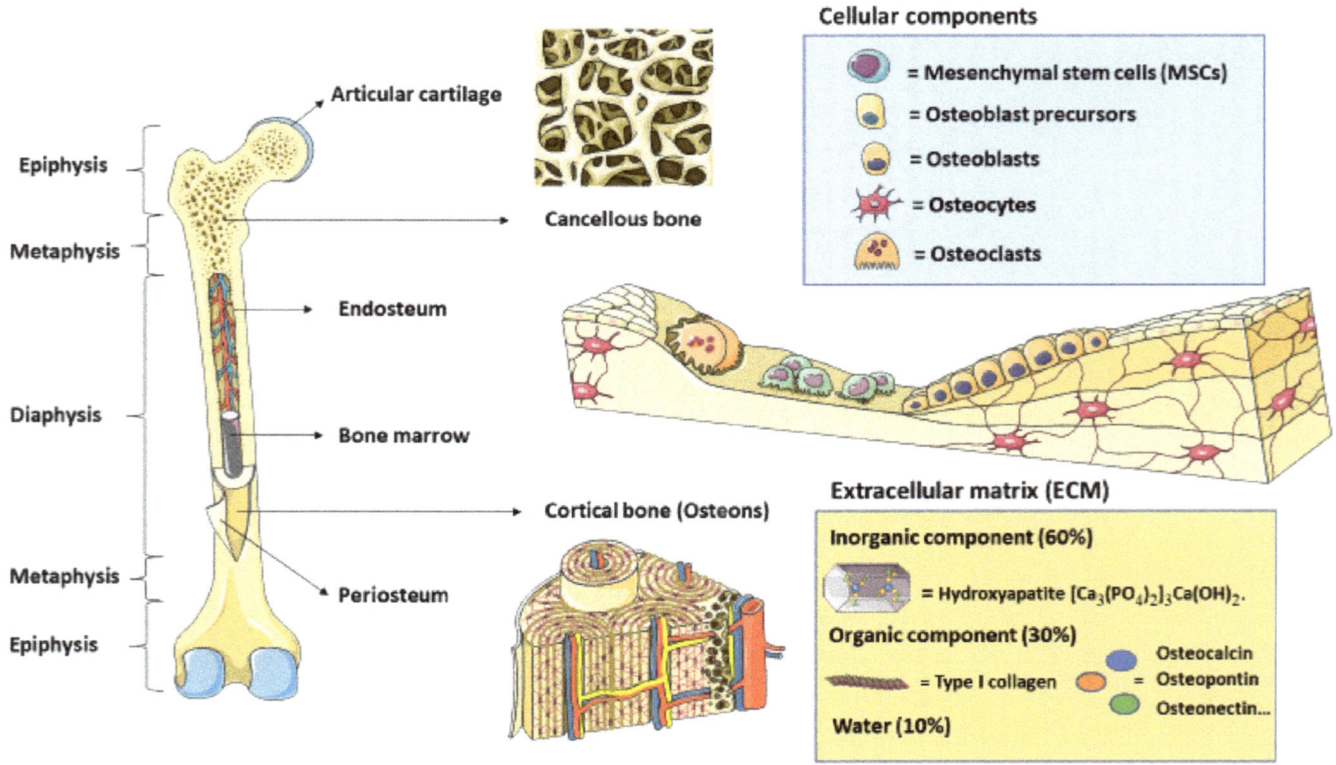

Fig. 5.3 This illustration presents a comprehensive view of bone anatomy, highlighting key regions, epiphysis, metaphysis, and diaphysis, and layers such as periosteum, cortical or cancellous bone, endosteum, and marrow. It also outlines bone histology, focusing on cells (e.g., stem cells, osteoblasts, osteocytes, osteoclasts) and extracellular matrix components like hydroxyapatite and collagen. Figure reproduced under license CC BY 4.0 [86] (https://creativecommons.org/licenses/by/4.0/)

have shown promise for enhancing bioactivity, immunomodulation, and angiogenesis. A notable example is a PLGA-PEG-PLGA triblock copolymer combined with 25% hydroxyapatite, which demonstrated shape-memory behavior and swelling-driven stabilization when inserted into femoral defects in rats. Additionally, PCL and PLGA-PEI scaffolds functionalized with BMPs have been shown to recruit stem cells in vivo, presenting a feasible cell-free option for treating non-load-bearing bone defects. These advancements underscore the value of 3D-printed polymer composites in current bone TE applications. Cartilage, in contrast to bone, is a soft tissue with unique biochemical and mechanical properties, displaying compositional gradients from the articular surface to the subchondral bone. It is composed predominantly of water (60–80%), type II collagen fibers, proteoglycans, chondrocytes, and varying levels of calcium ions. These features grant cartilage its tensile and compressive strength, as well as a high water retention capacity. However, its avascular, aneural, and alymphatic nature, coupled with a low cellular density, makes it particularly difficult to regenerate.

Cartilage TE requires softer substrates to promote chondrogenesis due to its pliable structure. Optimal pore sizes for cartilage scaffolds range between 90 and 120 μm, and compressive strengths of 0.5–3 MPa are considered adequate for functionality. Polymeric hydrogels are highly suitable due to their high water content and injectability [88]. Multilayered scaffolds with gradient compositions are particularly effective in replicating the interface between cartilage and subchondral bone. Similar to bone TE, cartilage regeneration involves modifying scaffold materials through coatings or blends to enhance performance. For instance, combining chitosan with PEG diacrylate improves both biocompatibility and mechanical characteristics, while PEG-based hydrogels have shown appropriate mechanical behavior for cartilage applications [89]. Furthermore, certain synthetic hydrogels such as polyacrylates with surface amine groups and poly(methyl methacrylate-co-methacrylic acid-co-PEG-diacrylate) have been reported to induce chondrogenesis in mesenchymal stem cells even without added growth factors. This effect is believed to be mediated by direct scaffold-cell interactions that stimulate endogenous expression of chondrogenic markers. Poly(L-lysine), for example, enhances chondrogenesis by upregulating N-cadherin when incorporated into oligo[poly(ethylene glycol)] fumarate hydrogels. The presence of accessible amine groups on scaffold surfaces is thus crucial for facilitating chondroinduction.

A recently developed 1,4-butanediol-based thermoplastic polyurethane elastomer has shown superior tribological properties for cartilage replacement compared to PCL and PLA. The scaffold's pore geometry, particularly when fabricated using FDM printing, significantly influenced cell behavior, with triangular pore designs promoting better MSC adhesion and proliferation [90]. While custom-designed polymers are being explored, commercially available thermoplastics like PCL and PLGA continue to be widely utilized for complex scaffold architectures, especially via 3D printing. The reproducibility and tunability of porous scaffolds made from these polymers make them especially attractive for mimicking the intricate structure of osteochondral tissues. 3D-printed gradient scaffolds incorporating osteogenic agents such as hydroxyapatite, tricalcium phosphate, decellularized ECM, or PCL conjugates with aggrecan-derived hyaluronic acid-binding peptides [90] are emerging as promising solutions to address cartilage degeneration and promote regeneration.

5.4.4 Corneal Regeneration

The human cornea resembles a fibril-reinforced laminate biocomposite in its transparency and mechanical resilience. It is a multilayered tissue comprising the epithelium, Bowman's layer, Descemet's membrane, endothelium, and predominantly the stroma, which makes up approximately 90% of the corneal thickness and contains collagen lamellae [91]. For tissue-engineered (TE) corneal scaffolds to be effective, they must emulate key characteristics of the native cornea, including (i) transparency, (ii) avascularity, (iii) minimal inflammatory response, (iv) mechanical properties suitable for suturing, and (v) sufficient nutrient permeability (~ 2.2×10^{-18} m^4 N^{-1} s^{-1}) [92]. Although collagen-based and decellularized scaffolds are the most widely utilized in corneal TE, collagen's natural origin also means it is expensive and mechanically fragile. In contrast, synthetic polymers have gained significant attention due to their favorable mechanical behavior, biocompatibility, and ease of processing, leading to their use in numerous preclinical studies and some clinical trials [93]. These polymers are also employed as carriers for limbal stem cells, particularly in contact lens form, to treat ocular surface damage and limbal stem cell deficiency.

The cornea's transparency primarily results from the uniformly spaced, nanoscale collagen fibrils in its extracellular matrix (ECM). Thus, scaffold alignment plays a crucial role in guiding stromal cell migration, orientation, and keratocyte phenotype expression. To replicate this, the chosen synthetic polymer must be compatible with advanced fabrication methods, such as electrospinning or 3D printing, which can generate aligned, curved, fibrous surfaces. However, achieving fiber diameters and spacing (~ 36 nm) similar to the natural stroma remains a fabrication challenge. Furthermore, scaffold curvature has been shown to influence both stromal and epithelial cell orientation and phenotype. Many synthetic polymers exhibit cloudiness due to their semicrystalline nature. Hence, amorphous polymers or scaffolds with adequate inter-fiber spacing are recommended to preserve transparency. Additionally, scaffold designs intended for use as contact lenses require sufficient softness and surface lubricity for wearer comfort. Synthetic polymers with long aliphatic chains and polar end groups typically exhibit the necessary softness, light hydrophilicity, and malleability for corneal TE.

Among synthetic polymers, polycaprolactone (PCL) has emerged as particularly promising. PCL is frequently combined with other polymers to enhance its degradation rate—such as poly(glycerol sebacate) (PGS), collagen, gelatin, chitosan, or ECM modifications often via electrospinning. While natural polymers like collagen offer high structural biomimicry, their high cost and mechanical limitations reduce their standalone applicability. Consequently, hybrid scaffolds combining synthetic and natural polymers have become a prevalent approach in engineering artificial corneas. These scaffold systems are anticipated to reduce reliance on human donor corneas and may even replace amniotic membranes commonly used in corneal stem cell transplants [94]. PCL's mechanical flexibility supports suturing, and its FDA-approved status enhances its suitability for biomedical use. For instance, Sun et al. fabricated corneal grafts using collagen and PCL with improved tensile strength. A specialized electrospinning technique also enabled the creation of hemispherical scaffolds from collagen and PCL, mimicking the natural cornea's radial alignment and curvature. These scaffolds showed enhanced corneal stem cell proliferation and upregulated relevant gene markers in vitro. Additionally, melt electrowriting has been applied to develop synthetic stromal substitutes using PCL. PGS, due to its amorphous and elastic properties, attributed to its chemical composition featuring long aliphatic chains and crosslinking, is especially suitable for corneal TE. When incorporated into aligned nanofibers, it improves hydrophilicity and promotes better cellular proliferation compared to PCL alone. The main goal of corneal TE is to reduce dependence on post-mortem donor tissue, which remains insufficient to meet global demand [95]. Given the cornea's relative anatomical simplicity, characterized by a lack of blood vessels and few cell types, tissue engineering holds considerable promise for revolutionizing the treatment of ocular diseases in the near future.

5.5 Synthetic Polymer TE Scaffolds with Clinical Applications

In cases where traditional medical treatments are no longer viable, tissue-engineered (TE) products incorporating synthetic polymer scaffolds have been employed for certain patients. Currently, a Phase II clinical trial is underway utilizing a tubular scaffold composed of electrospun polyglycolic acid (PGA) fibers and poly(caprolactone-co-lactide) [P(CL-co-LA)], seeded with autologous bone marrow-derived mononuclear cells, as a tissue-engineered vascular graft (TEVG) for managing complex congenital heart conditions in pediatric patients [96, 97]. Another ongoing TEVG clinical study involves a valved conduit fabricated from an electrospun scaffold made of polycaprolactone (PCL), polycarbonate (PC), and 2-ureido-4[1H]-pyrimidone (UPy). This scaffold, intended as an alternative to allograft conduits, which frequently fail in young children, has shown promising early outcomes in a limited patient group. Unlike the previous approach, this scaffold was designed to recruit the patient's endogenous cells without the addition of exogenous cells or bioactive agents. In these TEVG applications, the synthetic polymer plays a pivotal role in initiating tissue regeneration through a controlled foreign body response. As the polymer degrades, inflammation subsides and new tissue forms, highlighting the importance of both the degradation rate and modulation of the immune response in successful regeneration [98]. If degradation occurs too quickly, the scaffold may fail mechanically. Conversely, if degradation is too slow, a persistent foreign body reaction may arise, promoting fibrotic tissue buildup and impairing valve function. Thus, an optimal degradation timeline, slow and controlled, is crucial to enable proper tissue formation before the scaffold is fully resorbed. Additionally, modifying the scaffold's microstructure, alongside its chemical composition, is instrumental in maintaining the balance between tissue growth and scaffold degradation. Figure 5.4 represents an overview of diverse polymeric biomaterials uses across biomedical clinical applications.

Examples of synthetic polymer-based skin substitutes include Dermagraft and Trancyte, which are commercially available tissue-engineered dermal replacements [100]. These products leverage the structural simplicity and regenerative capacity of skin, as well as the extensive knowledge of skin cell biology. In Trancyte, fibroblasts are cultured on nylon scaffolds, whereas Dermagraft employs a polylactic acid (PLA)/PGA knitted scaffold in a bioreactor system. These scaffolds are made from commercially approved polymers and offer an advantage over collagen-based alternatives, as fibroblasts proliferate more readily on synthetic materials and deposit substantial extracellular matrix. Such products are used as cadaver skin alternatives in treating chronic wounds, including diabetic ulcers and severe burns. For cartilage regeneration, BioSeed-C represents a marketed TE product involving autologous cartilage

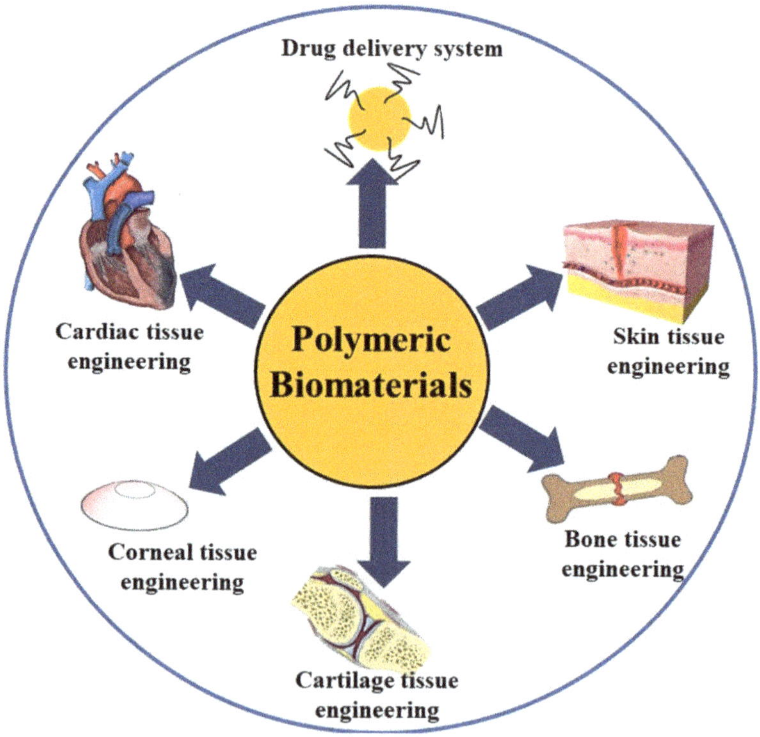

Fig. 5.4 Overview of diverse polymer uses across biomedical clinical applications. Figure reproduced under license CC BY 4.0 [99] (https://creativecommons.org/licenses/by/4.0/)

tissue engineering [101]. It features a scaffold composed of polylactic-co-glycolic acid (PLGA) and polydioxanone, seeded with autologous chondrocytes, which are later re-implanted into damaged cartilage. This approach has demonstrated significantly greater effectiveness than the traditional autologous chondrocyte implantation method [102]. In corneal epithelium repair, a clinical study has used silicone hydrogel contact lenses as carriers for autologous epithelial stem cells. At short- to mid-term follow-up, 63% of patients exhibited restored ocular surface integrity, suggesting this method is a promising alternative for treating limbal stem cell deficiency. While the current market offers only a limited number of synthetic polymer-based TE products, it is important to recognize that the field is still in its infancy. Despite the small number of available products, their demonstrated success is paving the way for broader development, regulatory standardization, and clinical acceptance. Moreover, these advancements are driving continued research, which will likely expand the scope of synthetic polymer applications in TE and improve therapeutic outcomes in other areas.

5.6 Conclusions

The advancement of innovative techniques and polymers with optimized properties remains essential in the ongoing development of biocompatible synthetic biomaterials. A key goal is to expand the availability of effective and safe tissue-engineered (TE) products for clinical applications. In addition to broader TE challenges—such as regulatory hurdles, difficulties in scaling up cell cultures, conducting clinical trials, and addressing vascularization issues—synthetic polymer-based TE faces specific barriers. These include the absence of standardized biocompatibility testing protocols and limitations in material selection due to incomplete knowledge of human biology, tissue-specific needs, and immune responses. To leverage the full potential of synthetic polymers, it is necessary to understand how their chemical composition interacts with host cells and the immune system during tissue regeneration. This requires collaboration among polymer scientists, bioengineers, clinicians, and biologists. Although recent decades have seen progress, achieving clinically viable, efficient, and affordable tissue regeneration remains a significant challenge. Given the ethical, financial, and logistical issues surrounding cell-based therapies, cell-free scaffolds offer a promising alternative for faster clinical adoption, placing polymers at the center of future TE strategies. There has been a significant increase in the synthesis and characterization of biodegradable synthetic polymers designed for scaffold applications in TE. Techniques like additive manufacturing and electrospinning, or their combination, are expected to remain dominant in scaffold fabrication [103]. Despite advances, discrepancies in how research is assessed—especially concerning biocompatibility—highlight the need for standardized evaluation methods across preclinical studies. Future TE developments are expected to include cell-free scaffolds that are easier to store, transport, and regulate. Instead of creating entirely new polymers, emphasis should be placed on tailoring existing materials to elicit favorable immune responses and promote regeneration. The lengthy and costly regulatory pathway for novel polymers may hinder their clinical translation, suggesting that new polymer development should be focused on niche applications where existing materials fall short. The evaluation of newly synthesized polymers should involve a critical analysis of existing options, identifying whether current limitations are understood and addressed, and whether performance benefits justify the regulatory burden.

Based on preclinical and clinical findings, the future use of synthetic polymers in TE varies by tissue type:

Soft Tissue: Efforts should focus on enhancing elasticity, tuning degradation rates, and mimicking native mechanical properties. Synthetic thermoplastic polyesters, their copolymers, and elastomers are expected to remain central materials. The development of cell-free scaffolds for in situ tissue regeneration will support broader clinical use. Heart Valves and Vessels: Biodegradable polyesters with prior FDA approval dominate current scaffold materials. The benefits of immunomodulatory, cell-free scaffolds are well-documented, and biofunctional scaffolds—either inherently antithrombogenic or functionalized with anticoagulant agents—are being explored. Further studies are needed to understand the interplay between TE heart valve (TEHV) stenosis, polymer properties, and inflammatory responses.

Muscle Tissue: Synthetic polymer-based elastic composites with micropatterns, electrical conductivity, or responsiveness to stimuli offer potential for mimicking muscle tissue. Additive manufacturing enables fabrication of aligned structures necessary for functional muscle regeneration. Electroconductive polymers that guide stem cell recruitment without the need for embedded cells are a focus. The development of biodegradable conductive polymers will significantly support advancements in muscle TE.

Nerve Tissue: Understanding how neurons respond to scaffold topography is essential. Improved regeneration is expected through the use of multichannel or nanostructured nerve conduits. Biodegradable conductive polymers also hold promise for bridging large nerve gaps and enhancing neural regeneration. Skin: Research should prioritize simpler, cell-free scaffold systems that mitigate issues such as distribution, preservation, and immunogenicity. The synergy of synthetic polymers with bioactive molecules is crucial. Polymers like polyvinylpyrrolidone (PVP), polycaprolactone (PCL), and poly(lactic-co-glycolic acid) (PLGA) are considered effective, safe, and cost-efficient when used with natural polymers to enhance cell adhesion.

Bone: Thermoplastic polyesters suitable for 3D printing complex scaffold structures are the preferred materials for bone TE. Scaffolds should support in situ osteogenesis and stem cell recruitment. PCL is frequently used due to its slow degradation rate and compatibility with 3D printing technologies.

Cartilage: Multilayered scaffolds or those with gradient compositions are needed to replicate osteochondral defects. Synthetic hydrogels are key for fabricating these scaffolds, particularly when combined with spatially controlled biochemical cues that eliminate the need for differentiation agents.

Cornea: Effective ocular TE requires scaffolds with radially aligned fibers and consistent cell availability. Enhancing understanding of how physical properties affect tissue repair is more impactful than synthesizing new polymers. Anti-inflammatory synthetic scaffolds are especially important for high-risk patients. Given the relatively lower clinical risk, corneal TE is anticipated to achieve clinical translation ahead of other tissue targets.

To support clinical application, safer in vivo testing protocols and reliable ex vivo evaluation methods are necessary. Overall, synthetic biocompatible polymers remain fundamental to the field of TE. Continued research into their interactions with human tissues and precise material control will enable the production of advanced biomaterials for TE, biomedical devices, and 3D-printed implants.

References

1. Boccaccini AR, Ma PX, Liverani L (2022) Tissue engineering using ceramics and polymers, vol 890
2. Ellahi A, Gupta S, Bose D, Chanda A (2025) A high-fidelity biomechanical modeling framework for injury prediction during frontal car crash. Comput Methods Biomech Biomed Eng 28:13–24
3. Afazal M, Gupta S, Tevatia A, Afreen S, Chanda A (2023) Computational fluid dynamics-based model for assessing rupture risk in cerebral arteries with varying aneurysm sizes. Computation 11:79
4. Gupta S, Gupta V, Chanda A (2022) Biomechanical modeling of novel high expansion auxetic skin grafts. Int J Numer Method Biomed Eng 38:e3586
5. Chanda A, Gupta S (2025) Healthcare entrepreneurship and management. Routledge, Taylor & Francis Group
6. Gupta S, Singh G, Chanda A (2021) Prediction of diabetic foot ulcer progression: a computational study. Biomed Phys Eng Express 7:065020
7. Gupta V, Singh G, Chanda A (2023) Modeling of metamaterial based incision patterns for generating high expansions in skin grafts. Clin Biomech 110:106118
8. Singh G, Chanda A (2022) Biomechanical modeling of progressive wound healing: a computational study. Biomed Eng Adv 4:100055
9. Yadav P, Kamboj M, Das B (2024) Application of nanotechnology in antimicrobial coating on surgical instruments. In: Applications of nanotechnology in biomedical engineering, pp 150–168. https://doi.org/10.1201/9781003432661-9
10. Ali SAM, Zhong SP, Doherty PJ, Williams DF (1993) Mechanisms of polymer degradation in implantable devices. I. Poly(caprolactone). Biomaterials 14:648–656
11. Bernard M, Jubeli E, Pungente MD, Yagoubi N (2018) Biocompatibility of polymer-based biomaterials and medical devices—regulations, in vitro screening and risk-management. Biomater Sci 6:2025–2053
12. Verma S, Singh G, Chanda A (2024) Development of a computational framework for determination of detrimental vibrations on the human spine segments. Multiscale Sci Eng 6(1):48–56
13. Verma S, Singh G, Chanda A (2023) A novel finite element model for the study of harmful vibrations on the aging spine. Computation 11:93
14. Pappalardo D, Mathisen T, Finne-Wistrand A (2019) Biocompatibility of resorbable polymers: a historical perspective and framework for the future. Biomacromolecules 20:1465–1477
15. Singh G, Yadav P, Chanda A (2024) Development of biofidelic skin simulants based on fresh cadaveric skin tests. Eur Burn J 5:454–463

16. Yadav P et al (2025) Gelatin multiwalled carbon nanotube composite 3D printed semi biological mesh for abdominal hernia treatment. Chem Asian J 20:e202401136
17. Smits AIPM, Bouten CVC (2018) Tissue engineering meets immunoengineering: prospective on personalized in situ tissue engineering strategies. Curr Opin Biomed Eng 6:17–26
18. Verma S, Chanda A (2024) State-of-the-art of finite element modelling of the human spine to study the impact of vibrations: a review. Int J Comput Methods Eng Sci Mech 25:225–247
19. Camarero-Espinosa S et al (2022) 3D printed dual-porosity scaffolds: the combined effect of stiffness and porosity in the modulation of macrophage polarization. Adv Healthc Mater 11:e2101415
20. Singh G, Chanda A (2024) Biofidelic gallbladder tissue surrogates. Adv Mater Process Technol. https://doi.org/10.1080/2374068X.2023.2198835
21. Afazal M, Afreen S, Chanda A (2023) Computational modelling and analysis of hard tissue behavior around 0.5 mm and 0.85 mm platform switched abutment using 3D finite element analysis. Forces Mech 13:100243
22. Rothschild BM et al (2023) Design, manufacturing, and trial of a 3D printed customized finger splint for patients with rheumatoid arthritis. Rheumato 3:51–62
23. Woodruff MA, Hutmacher DW (2010) The return of a forgotten polymer—polycaprolactone in the 21st century. Prog Polym Sci 35:1217–1256
24. Palmer JA, Abberton KM, Mitchell GM, Morrison WA (2014) Macrophage phenotype in response to implanted synthetic scaffolds: an immunohistochemical study in the rat. Cells Tissues Organs 199:169–183
25. Luo L et al (2016) Polycaprolactone nanofibrous mesh reduces foreign body reaction and induces adipose flap expansion in tissue engineering chamber. Int J Nanomed 11:6471–6483
26. Bose D, Gupta S, Chanda A (2025) Scalable direct manufacturing of a functional multipurpose wrist-hand orthosis using 3D printing. Ann 3D Print Med 17:100186
27. Chanda A, Gupta V, Gupta S (2024) Development and mechanical testing of auxetic incisions on human cadaveric skin, pp 89–99. https://doi.org/10.1007/978-981-97-4383-4_7
28. Lin X et al (2017) Hyaluronic acid coating enhances biocompatibility of nonwoven PGA scaffold and cartilage formation. Tissue Eng Part C Methods 23:86–97
29. Yassin MA et al (2019) 3D and porous RGDC-functionalized polyester-based scaffolds as a niche to induce osteogenic differentiation of human bone marrow stem cells. Macromol Biosci 19:1900049
30. Jain S et al (2021) Understanding of how the properties of medical grade lactide based copolymer scaffolds influence adipose tissue regeneration: sterilization and a systematic in vitro assessment. Mater Sci Eng C 124:112020
31. Wissing TB, Bonito V, Bouten CVC, Smits AIPM (2017) Biomaterial-driven in situ cardiovascular tissue engineering—a multi-disciplinary perspective. npj Regen Med 2(1):1–20
32. Naureen B, Haseeb ASMA, Basirun WJ, Muhamad F (2021) Recent advances in tissue engineering scaffolds based on polyurethane and modified polyurethane. Mater Sci Eng C 118:111228
33. Xu C, Huang Y, Tang L, Hong Y (2017) Low-initial-modulus biodegradable polyurethane elastomers for soft tissue regeneration. ACS Appl Mater Interfaces 9:2169–2180
34. Mi HY et al (2017) Biocompatible, degradable thermoplastic polyurethane based on polycaprolactone-block-polytetrahydrofuran-block-polycaprolactone copolymers for soft tissue engineering. J Mater Chem B 5:4137–4151
35. Jiang C et al (2021) Self-healing polyurethane-elastomer with mechanical tunability for multiple biomedical applications in vivo. Nat Commun 12(1):1–13
36. Tran RT, Yang J, Ameer GA (2015) Citrate-based biomaterials and their applications in regenerative engineering. Annu Rev Mater Res 45:277–310
37. Van Beek DJM, Gillissen MAJ, Van As BAC, Palmans ARA, Sijbesma RP (2007) Supramolecular copolyesters with tunable properties. Macromolecules 40:6340–6348
38. Piluso S et al (2021) 3D bioprinting of molecularly engineered PEG-based hydrogels utilizing gelatin fragments. Biofabrication 13:045008

39. Morris VB, Nimbalkar S, Younesi M, McClellan P, Akkus O (2017) Mechanical properties, cytocompatibility and manufacturability of chitosan: PEGDA hybrid-gel scaffolds by stereolithography. Ann Biomed Eng 45:286–296
40. Rasines Mazo A et al (2020) Ring opening polymerization of α-amino acids: advances in synthesis, architecture and applications of polypeptides and their hybrids. Chem Soc Rev 49:4737–4834
41. Shirbin SJ, Karimi F, Chan NJA, Heath DE, Qiao GG (2016) Macroporous hydrogels composed entirely of synthetic polypeptides: biocompatible and enzyme biodegradable 3D cellular scaffolds. Biomacromolecules 17:2981–2991
42. Jiménez G et al (2019) A soft 3D polyacrylate hydrogel recapitulates the cartilage niche and allows growth-factor free tissue engineering of human articular cartilage. Acta Biomater 90:146–156
43. Chanda A, Ruchti T, Unnikrishnan V (2018) Computational modeling of wound suture: a review. IEEE Rev Biomed Eng 11:165–176
44. Singh G, Chanda A (2024) Development and biomechanical testing of artificial surrogates for vaginal tissue. Adv Mater Process Technol. https://doi.org/10.1080/2374068X.2023.2198837
45. Gupta V, Singh G, Chanda A (2023) Development of hierarchical auxetic skin graft simulants with high expansion potential. Biomed Eng Adv 5:100087
46. Chen H, Yuan L, Song W, Wu Z, Li D (2008) Biocompatible polymer materials: role of protein–surface interactions. Prog Polym Sci 33:1059–1087
47. Jurak M, Wiącek AE, Ładniak A, Przykaza K, Szafran K (2021) What affects the biocompatibility of polymers? Adv Colloid Interface Sci 294:102451
48. Singh G, Gupta V, Chanda A (2022) Artificial skin with varying biomechanical properties. Mater Today Proc 62:3162–3166
49. Gupta V, Chanda A (2023) Biomechanical modelling of hierarchical metamaterials for skin grafting. In: Materials horizons: from nature to nanomaterials (part F1471), pp 71–83
50. Saltzman WM, Kyriakides TR (2014) Cell interactions with polymers. In: Principles of tissue engineering, 4th edn, pp 385–406. https://doi.org/10.1016/B978-0-12-398358-9.00020-3
51. Mondschein RJ, Kanitkar A, Williams CB, Verbridge SS, Long TE (2017) Polymer structure-property requirements for stereolithographic 3D printing of soft tissue engineering scaffolds. Biomaterials 140:170–188
52. Wandel MB et al (2021) Concomitant control of mechanical properties and degradation in resorbable elastomer-like materials using stereochemistry and stoichiometry for soft tissue engineering. Nat Commun 12(1):1–13
53. Gupta V, Chanda A (2023) Auxetic incisions with alternating slit shapes: a promising technique for enhancing synthetic skin grafts expansion. Mater Res Express 10:075802
54. Gupta V, Gupta S, Chanda A (2023) Development of an ultra-low-cost planar biaxial tester for soft tissue characterization. Biomed Phys Eng Express 9:025011
55. Jiang C et al (2022) Biomechanics of skin grafts: effect of pattern size, spacing and orientation. Eng Res Express 4:015006
56. Kim WJ, Kim M, Kim GH (2018) 3D-printed biomimetic scaffold simulating microfibril muscle structure. Adv Funct Mater 28:1800405
57. Ge J et al (2021) Engineering conductive antioxidative antibacterial nanocomposite hydrogel scaffolds with oriented channels promotes structure-functional skeletal muscle regeneration. Chem Eng J 425:130333
58. Beldjilali-Labro M et al (2018) Biomaterials in tendon and skeletal muscle tissue engineering: current trends and challenges. Materials 11:1116
59. Ju YM, Choi JS, Atala A, Yoo JJ, Lee SJ (2010) Bilayered scaffold for engineering cellularized blood vessels. Biomaterials 31:4313–4321
60. De Kort BJ et al (2021) Inflammatory and regenerative processes in bioresorbable synthetic pulmonary valves up to two years in sheep–spatiotemporal insights augmented by Raman microspectroscopy. Acta Biomater 135:243–259

61. Singh G, Chanda A (2024) Finite element modeling of diabetic foot: a state-of-the-art review. Eng Res Express 6:012507
62. Chhikara K, Sidhu SS, Gupta S, Saharawat S, Kataria C, Chanda A (2023) Development and effectiveness testing of a novel 3D-printed multi-material orthosis in nurses with plantar foot pain. Prosthesis 5:73–87
63. Chhikara K, Gupta S, Bose D, Kataria C, Chanda A (2023) Development and trial of a multipurpose customized orthosis for activities of daily living in patients with spinal cord injury. Prosthesis 5:467–479
64. Kluin J et al (2017) In situ heart valve tissue engineering using a bioresorbable elastomeric implant—from material design to 12 months follow-up in sheep. Biomaterials 125:101–117
65. Amani H, Kazerooni H, Hassanpoor H, Akbarzadeh A, Pazoki-Toroudi H (2019) Tailoring synthetic polymeric biomaterials towards nerve tissue engineering: a review. Artif Cells Nanomed Biotechnol 47:3524–3539
66. Ioannidis K et al (2020) A custom ultra-low-cost 3D bioprinter supports cell growth and differentiation. Front Bioeng Biotechnol 8:580889
67. Doblado LR, Martínez-Ramos C, Pradas MM (2021) Biomaterials for neural tissue engineering. Front Nanotechnol 3:643507
68. Asplund M, Nyberg T, Inganäs O (2010) Electroactive polymers for neural interfaces. Polym Chem 1:1374–1391
69. Yannas IV, Burke JF (1980) Design of an artificial skin. I. Basic design principles. J Biomed Mater Res 14:339–339
70. Chhikara K, Gupta S, Chanda A (2022) Development of a novel foot orthosis for plantar pain reduction. Mater Today Proc 62:3532–3537
71. Chanda A, Flynn Z, Unnikrishnan V (2018) Biomechanical characterization of normal and prolapsed vaginal tissue surrogates. J Mech Med Biol 18:1750100
72. Chanda A, Chatterjee S, Gupta V (2020) Soft composite based hyperelastic model for anisotropic tissue characterization. J Compos Mater 54:4525–4534
73. Klimek K, Ginalska G (2020) Proteins and peptides as important modifiers of the polymer scaffolds for tissue engineering applications—a review. Polymers 12:844
74. Xu R et al (2023) Recent advances in biodegradable and biocompatible synthetic polymers used in skin wound healing. Materials 16:5459
75. Review on electrospun nanofibers scaffold and biomedical applications. https://www.researchgate.net/publication/268261967_Review_on_Electrospun_Nanofibers_Scaffold_and_Biomedical_Applications
76. Chanda A, Upchurch W (2018) Biomechanical modeling of wounded skin. J Compos Sci 2:69
77. Gupta V, Chanda A (2021) Expansion potential of skin grafts with novel I-shaped auxetic incisions. Biomed Phys Eng Express 8:015016
78. Chanda A, Unnikrishnan V, Flynn Z, Lackey K (2017) Experimental study on tissue phantoms to understand the effect of injury and suturing on human skin mechanical properties. Proc Inst Mech Eng Part H J Eng Med 231:80–91
79. Wu K, Wu X, Guo J, Jiao Y, Zhou C (2021) Facile polyphenol–europium assembly enabled functional poly(L-lactic acid) nanofiber mats with enhanced antioxidation and angiogenesis for accelerated wound healing. Adv Healthc Mater 10:2100793
80. Gupta V, Singla R, Chanda A (2023) Development and characterization of novel anisotropic skin graft simulants. Dermato 3:114–130
81. Gupta V, Chanda A (2024) Mechanical characterization of alternating slit, I-shaped and rotating triangle based auxetic skin graft phantoms. Mech Adv Mater Struct. https://doi.org/10.1080/15376494.2023.2250782
82. Gupta V, Singh G, Gupta S, Chanda A (2023) Expansion potential of auxetic prosthetic skin grafts: a review. Eng Res Express 5:022003
83. Zhang B, Huang J, Narayan RJ (2020) Gradient scaffolds for osteochondral tissue engineering and regeneration. J Mater Chem B 8:8149–8170

84. Ogueri KS et al (2021) In vivo evaluation of the regenerative capability of glycylglycine ethyl ester-substituted polyphosphazene and poly(lactic-co-glycolic acid) blends: a rabbit critical-sized bone defect model. ACS Biomater Sci Eng 7:1564–1572
85. Chanda A (2018) Biomechanical modeling of human skin tissue surrogates. Biomimetics 3:18
86. Fraile-Martínez O et al (2021) Applications of polymeric composites in bone tissue engineering and jawbone regeneration. Polymers 13:3429
87. Kondiah PPD et al (2020) Recent progress in 3D-printed polymeric scaffolds for bone tissue engineering. In: Advanced 3D-printed systems and nanosystems for drug delivery and tissue engineering, pp 59–81. https://doi.org/10.1016/B978-0-12-818471-4.00003-0
88. Lam J et al (2016) Evaluation of cell-laden polyelectrolyte hydrogels incorporating poly(L-lysine) for applications in cartilage tissue engineering. Biomaterials 83:332–346
89. Wang J, Zhang F, Tsang WP, Wan C, Wu C (2017) Fabrication of injectable high strength hydrogel based on 4-arm star PEG for cartilage tissue engineering. Biomaterials 120:11–21
90. Martínez-Moreno D et al (2021) Pore geometry influences growth and cell adhesion of infrapatellar mesenchymal stem cells in biofabricated 3D thermoplastic scaffolds useful for cartilage tissue engineering. Mater Sci Eng C 122:111933
91. Mobaraki M et al (2019) Corneal repair and regeneration: current concepts and future directions. Front Bioeng Biotechnol 7
92. Etebu E (2013) Mechanical and rheological characterization of the cornea
93. Mahdavi SS, Abdekhodaie MJ, Mashayekhan S, Baradaran-Rafii A, Djalilian AR (2020) Bioengineering approaches for corneal regenerative medicine. Tissue Eng Regen Med 17:567–593
94. Ramachandran C et al (2019) Synthetic biodegradable alternatives to the use of the amniotic membrane for corneal regeneration: assessment of local and systemic toxicity in rabbits. Br J Ophthalmol 103:286–292
95. Baird PN, Machin H, Brown KD (2021) Corneal supply and the use of technology to reduce its demand: a review. Clin Exp Ophthalmol 49:1078–1090
96. Drews JD et al (2020) Spontaneous reversal of stenosis in tissue-engineered vascular grafts. Sci Transl Med 12
97. Two-year study of the safety and efficacy of the second-generation tissue engineered vascular grafts. Clinical Research Trial Listing. https://www.centerwatch.com/clinical-trials/listings/NCT04467671/two-year-study-of-the-safety-and-efficacy-of-the-second-generation-tissue-engineered-vascular-grafts
98. de Kort BJ et al (2021) Immuno-regenerative biomaterials for in situ cardiovascular tissue engineering—do patient characteristics warrant precision engineering? Adv Drug Deliv Rev 178:113960
99. Kalirajan C, Dukle A, Nathanael AJ, Oh TH, Manivasagam G (2021) A critical review on polymeric biomaterials for biomedical applications. Polymers 13:3015
100. Kumar RJ, Kimble RM, Boots R, Pegg SP (2004) Treatment of partial-thickness burns: a prospective, randomized trial using Transcyte™. ANZ J Surg 74:622–626
101. BioSeed®-C repairs knee cartilage effectively (2007) Nat Clin Pract Rheumatol 3(7):371
102. Ossendorf C et al (2007) Treatment of posttraumatic and focal osteoarthritic cartilage defects of the knee with autologous polymer-based three-dimensional chondrocyte grafts: 2-year clinical results. Arthritis Res Ther 9:R41
103. Ma J et al (2021) Recent trends in therapeutic strategies for repairing endometrial tissue in intrauterine adhesion. Biomater Res 25:40

Chapter 6
Biocomposites-Based Artificial Tissues

6.1 Introduction

6.1.1 Definition and Concept of Biocomposites

Biocomposites are composite materials formed by combining a matrix (resin) with reinforcement materials derived from natural sources. In the context of tissue engineering, biocomposites are designed to mimic the structural and functional properties of native tissues, facilitating the repair or replacement of damaged biological structures. The matrix in biocomposites can be composed of biodegradable polymers such as polylactic acid (PLA), polycaprolactone (PCL), or poly(lactic-co-glycolic acid) (PLGA), which provide a supportive environment for cell attachment and proliferation. The reinforcement phase often includes natural fibers like collagen, chitosan, or hydroxyapatite (HA), which enhance the mechanical strength and bioactivity of the composite. For instance, bone is a natural composite consisting of collagen fibers reinforced with HA crystals, providing both flexibility and rigidity essential for load-bearing functions [1]. The integration of natural and synthetic components in biocomposites allows for the tailoring of properties such as degradation rate, mechanical strength, and biocompatibility. This customization is crucial for developing scaffolds that can support tissue regeneration while gradually degrading to be replaced by native tissue. Moreover, the use of natural fibers contributes to the sustainability and environmental friendliness of biocomposites, aligning with the growing emphasis on green materials in biomedical applications. Biocomposites in tissue engineering represent a synergistic approach that combines the advantageous properties of natural and synthetic materials to create scaffolds that support tissue regeneration, offering a promising avenue for advancing regenerative medicine [2].

A. Chanda and D. Sharma, *Handbook of Artificial Tissues, Biofabrication and Bioprinting, Volume I*, Biomedical Materials for Multi-functional Applications,
https://doi.org/10.1007/978-981-92-1307-8_6

6.1.2 History of Biocomposites in Medicine

The application of biocomposites in medicine has evolved significantly over the past century, with early efforts focusing on developing materials that could integrate with biological tissues without eliciting adverse reactions. In the 1940s, researchers began exploring the use of metals like titanium and tantalum for implants due to their favorable mechanical properties and biocompatibility. Notably, Gerald Louis Burke conducted pioneering work in analyzing and fabricating tantalum for orthopedic and dental implants, demonstrating its ability to bond with living tissue. A significant milestone was achieved in the late 1960s when Larry L. Hench developed Bioglass 45S5, the first bioactive glass capable of forming a bond with bone tissue. This innovation marked the inception of bioceramics and opened new possibilities for creating materials that could actively participate in the healing process. The concept of osseointegration, introduced by Per-Ingvar Brånemark in the 1950s, further advanced the field by demonstrating the potential for titanium implants to integrate directly with bone, leading to the development of modern dental and orthopedic implants. Over the years, the integration of natural polymers with synthetic materials has led to the development of advanced biocomposites that offer improved mechanical properties and biocompatibility. These materials have been employed in various medical applications, including bone grafts, dental restorations, and tissue engineering scaffolds, reflecting the ongoing evolution and significance of biocomposites in medicine [3].

6.1.3 Importance of Biocomposites for Artificial Tissues

The development of artificial tissues necessitates materials that can replicate the complex mechanical and biological properties of native tissues. Biocomposites play a crucial role in this endeavor by offering customizable properties that can be tailored to meet specific tissue requirements. One of the primary advantages of biocomposites is their ability to combine the strength and durability of synthetic polymers with the bioactivity and biocompatibility of natural materials. For example, incorporating hydroxyapatite into polymer matrices can enhance osteoconductivity, promoting bone tissue regeneration. Moreover, the structural characteristics of biocomposites, such as porosity and pore interconnectivity, are critical for facilitating cell infiltration, nutrient diffusion, and vascularization, all of which are essential for successful tissue regeneration. Advanced fabrication techniques, including 3D printing and electrospinning, allow for precise control over these structural features, enabling the creation of scaffolds that closely mimic the architecture of native tissues [4]. Biocomposites also offer the potential for controlled degradation, ensuring that the scaffold provides temporary support while gradually being replaced by newly formed tissue. This degradation must be carefully balanced to match the rate of tissue regeneration, avoiding premature loss of mechanical support or prolonged presence that could

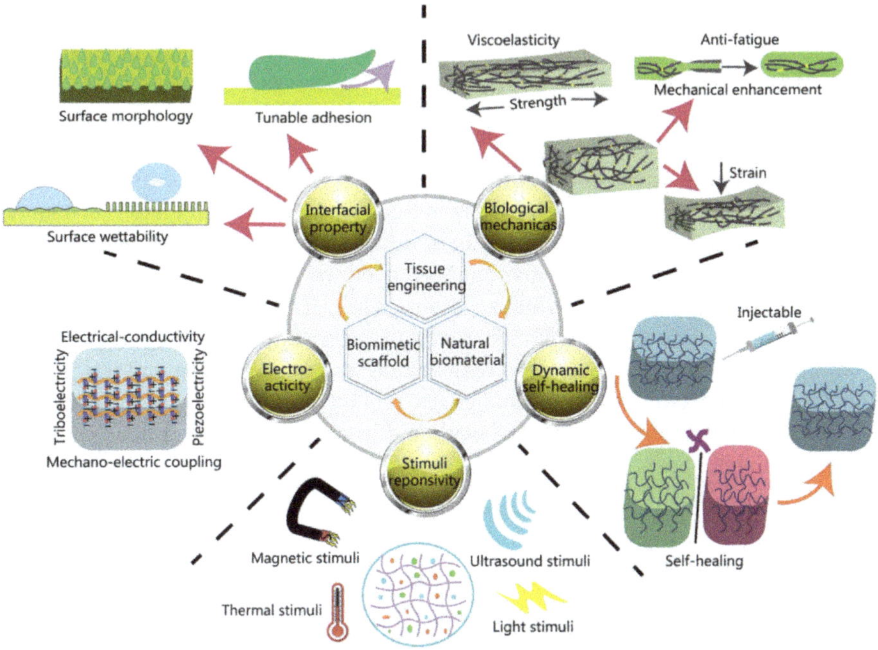

Fig. 6.1 Strategic design and fabrication of biomimetic natural biomaterials (BNBMs) endowed with specific characteristics. Figure reproduced under license CC BY 4.0 [6] (https://creativecommons.org/licenses/by/4.0/)

impede healing [5]. Biocomposites are integral to the advancement of artificial tissues in regenerative medicine. Their customizable properties, biocompatibility, and ability to support tissue regeneration make them indispensable in developing effective and functional tissue-engineered constructions. Figure 6.1 illustrates the strategic design and fabrication of biomimetic natural biomaterials (BNBMs) endowed with specific characteristics that replicate the properties of the native extracellular matrix (ECM) of tissues.

6.2 Classification of Biocomposites

6.2.1 Natural-Natural Biocomposites: Collagen-Hydroxyapatite Composites for Bone Repair

Natural-natural biocomposites are composed entirely of naturally derived components, aiming to replicate the complex architecture and functionality of native tissues. A quintessential example is the collagen-hydroxyapatite (Col-HA) composite, extensively utilized in bone tissue engineering. Collagen, the primary structural protein in the extracellular matrix, provides excellent biocompatibility and biodegradability and promotes cell adhesion and proliferation. Hydroxyapatite (HA), a naturally occurring mineral form of calcium apatite, contributes rigidity and osteoconductivity, essential for bone regeneration. The integration of collagen and HA results in a composite that closely mimics the composition and mechanical properties of natural bone. The fabrication of Col-HA composites involves techniques such as co-precipitation, freeze-drying, and electrospinning, allowing control over porosity and mechanical strength. These scaffolds support osteoblast attachment, proliferation, and differentiation, facilitating new bone formation. Moreover, the biodegradability of collagen ensures gradual replacement by native tissue, while HA provides long-term structural support [7]. Studies have demonstrated the efficacy of Col-HA composites in repairing critical-sized bone defects, with enhanced vascularization and mineralization observed in vivo. However, challenges remain in optimizing the mechanical properties to match those of cortical bone and in ensuring uniform distribution of HA within the collagen matrix [8].

6.2.2 Natural-Synthetic Biocomposites: Chitosan-Poly(Lactic Acid) (PLA) Composites for Soft Tissues

Natural-synthetic biocomposites combine naturally derived polymers with synthetic materials to harness the advantages of both. Chitosan, obtained from the deacetylation of chitin, offers biocompatibility, biodegradability, and antimicrobial properties. Poly(lactic acid) (PLA), a synthetic aliphatic polyester, provides mechanical strength and controlled degradation rates. The amalgamation of chitosan and PLA results in composites suitable for soft tissue engineering applications, such as skin, cartilage, and vascular tissues. These composites exhibit improved mechanical properties, enhanced cell adhesion, and controlled degradation profiles. Fabrication methods include solvent casting, electrospinning, and 3D printing, allowing the creation of scaffolds with tailored porosity and architecture. Research indicates that chitosan-PLA composites support fibroblast proliferation and extracellular matrix deposition, essential for soft tissue regeneration. Furthermore, the antimicrobial properties of chitosan reduce the risk of infection at the implantation site. However, optimizing the ratio of chitosan to PLA is crucial to balance mechanical strength and degradation rates [9].

6.2.3 *Synthetic-Synthetic Biocomposites: Poly(Lactic-co-Glycolic Acid) (PLGA) with Hydroxyapatite*

Synthetic-synthetic biocomposites consist entirely of synthetic materials, offering precise control over composition, degradation rates, and mechanical properties. A prominent example is the combination of poly(lactic-co-glycolic acid) (PLGA) with hydroxyapatite (HA), extensively researched for bone tissue engineering. PLGA is a biodegradable copolymer approved by the FDA for various biomedical applications. Its degradation rate can be tailored by adjusting the lactic to glycolic acid ratio. Incorporating HA into PLGA matrices enhances osteoconductivity and mechanical strength, making the composite suitable for load-bearing bone defects. Fabrication techniques such as solvent casting, particulate leaching, and 3D printing enable the creation of porous scaffolds with interconnected pores, facilitating cell infiltration and nutrient diffusion. Studies have shown that PLGA-HA composites support osteoblast adhesion, proliferation, and differentiation, leading to effective bone regeneration. However, challenges include potential acidic degradation products from PLGA, which may affect local pH and biocompatibility.

6.2.4 *Functionalized Biocomposites: Biocomposites with Bioactive Molecules or Growth Factors*

Functionalized biocomposites are engineered to incorporate bioactive molecules, such as growth factors, peptides, or drugs, to enhance biological responses and tissue regeneration. These composites aim to provide not only structural support but also biochemical cues to guide cell behavior. Incorporation of growth factors like bone morphogenetic proteins (BMPs), vascular endothelial growth factor (VEGF), or transforming growth factor-beta (TGF-β) into biocomposites has shown to accelerate tissue healing processes. Delivery methods include physical adsorption, covalent bonding, or encapsulation within nanoparticles embedded in the scaffold matrix. Functionalized biocomposites have demonstrated enhanced angiogenesis, osteogenesis, and neurogenesis in various tissue engineering applications. For instance, scaffolds releasing BMP-2 have shown improved bone regeneration, while VEGF-loaded scaffolds promote vascularization in engineered tissues. Challenges in this domain involve achieving controlled and sustained release of bioactive agents and maintaining their stability and activity during scaffold fabrication and implantation [10].

6.3 Properties of Biocomposites for Artificial Tissues

6.3.1 Mechanical Properties: Flexibility, Strength, and Durability of Biocomposites

Mechanical properties are critical in designing biocomposites for artificial tissues, ensuring that the materials can withstand physiological loads and stresses. Flexibility, strength, and durability are paramount to mimic the native tissue's mechanical behavior and to maintain structural integrity during tissue regeneration. Flexibility in biocomposites allows them to conform to the dynamic movements of the body, which is essential for soft tissue applications. Materials such as polycaprolactone (PCL) exhibit significant flexibility, making them suitable for applications like vascular grafts and nerve conduits [11]. The incorporation of natural polymers like gelatin can further enhance the flexibility and elasticity of the composite, closely resembling the mechanical properties of native tissues. Strength is another vital parameter, especially for load-bearing applications such as bone and cartilage repair. The addition of inorganic fillers like hydroxyapatite (HA) to polymer matrices has been shown to improve the compressive strength of biocomposites, making them more suitable for orthopedic applications [12]. Moreover, the alignment of reinforcing fibers within the composite can significantly enhance tensile strength, providing resistance against mechanical deformation. Durability ensures that the biocomposite maintains its mechanical integrity over the required period for tissue regeneration. This involves resistance to fatigue, wear, and degradation under physiological conditions. Studies have demonstrated that crosslinking strategies and the use of high-molecular-weight polymers can improve the durability of biocomposites, ensuring sustained performance during the healing process. Tailoring the mechanical properties of biocomposites through material selection and structural design is crucial for their successful application in tissue engineering.

6.3.2 Biocompatibility and Bioactivity: Interaction with Cells and Tissues

Biocompatibility and bioactivity are essential properties of biocomposites, determining their ability to interact favorably with biological systems. Biocompatibility ensures that the material does not elicit an adverse immune response, while bioactivity refers to the material's ability to elicit specific biological responses, such as promoting cell adhesion, proliferation, and differentiation. The initial interaction between biocomposites and the biological environment involves protein adsorption onto the material's surface. This protein layer mediates subsequent cell attachment and signaling. Studies have shown that the surface chemistry and topography of biocomposites significantly influence protein adsorption patterns, thereby affecting cell behavior [13]. Bioactive biocomposites can be engineered to release growth factors or other signaling molecules that promote tissue regeneration. For instance, incorporating bone morphogenetic proteins (BMPs) into biocomposites has been demonstrated to enhance osteogenic differentiation and bone formation [14]. Moreover, the degradation products of biocomposites should be non-toxic and easily metabolized or excreted by the body. Ensuring biocompatibility and bioactivity is thus a multifaceted approach involving material selection, surface modification, and controlled degradation [15].

6.3.3 *Degradability and Biodegradability: Controlled Breakdown for Tissue Regeneration*

Degradability and biodegradability are pivotal properties in biocomposite design, enabling the material to break down at a rate that matches tissue regeneration. Controlled degradation ensures that the scaffold provides temporary support while being replaced by native tissue over time [16]. Biodegradation involves the breakdown of materials through biological processes, often mediated by enzymes or hydrolysis. Polymers like polylactic acid (PLA) and polycaprolactone (PCL) are commonly used in biocomposites due to their predictable degradation profiles [17]. The degradation rate can be tailored by modifying the polymer's molecular weight, crystallinity, or by copolymerization. The byproducts of degradation should be non-toxic and should not elicit an inflammatory response. For example, PLA degrades into lactic acid, which is naturally metabolized by the body. However, accumulation of acidic degradation products can lead to localized pH changes, potentially affecting cell viability. Therefore, incorporating buffering agents or designing composites with neutral degradation products is essential [12, 18]. The degradability of biocomposites must be carefully engineered to align with the specific tissue regeneration timeline, ensuring optimal integration and function.

6.3.4 *Surface Properties and Porosity: Impact on Cell Attachment and Proliferation*

The surface properties and porosity of biocomposites significantly influence cell attachment, proliferation, and overall tissue integration. Surface characteristics such as roughness, hydrophilicity, and chemical functionality determine protein adsorption and subsequent cell behavior [19]. Surface roughness at the micro- and nanoscale can enhance cell adhesion by providing more anchoring points. For instance, increasing the surface roughness of titanium implants has been shown to improve osteoblast attachment and proliferation. Similarly, hydrophilic surfaces promote better protein adsorption and cell spreading compared to hydrophobic ones.

Porosity is crucial for nutrient diffusion, waste removal, and vascularization within the scaffold. An interconnected porous network allows for cell infiltration and tissue ingrowth. Optimal pore sizes vary depending on the target tissue; for bone tissue engineering, pore sizes between 100 and 500 μm are considered ideal. Moreover, the fabrication method can influence the porosity and surface properties of the biocomposite. Techniques like freeze-drying, electrospinning, and 3D printing allow for precise control over scaffold architecture, enabling the design of structures that closely mimic the extracellular matrix. The surface properties and porosity of biocomposites are essential to facilitate cell attachment, proliferation, and successful tissue regeneration.

6.4 Applications of Biocomposites in Artificial Tissue Engineering

6.4.1 Cartilage and Soft Tissue Engineering: Flexibility and Elasticity in Cartilage Repair

Articular cartilage is a specialized connective tissue that provides a smooth, lubricated surface for joint movement and distributes mechanical loads. Due to its avascular nature and limited regenerative capacity, cartilage injuries often lead to degenerative diseases like osteoarthritis. Biocomposites have emerged as promising materials for cartilage repair, offering tailored mechanical properties and biological functionalities. Natural polymers such as collagen, chitosan, and hyaluronic acid have been extensively studied for cartilage tissue engineering. Collagen, the primary structural protein in cartilage, provides a supportive matrix for cell attachment and proliferation. Chitosan, derived from chitin, exhibits biocompatibility and biodegradability, promoting chondrocyte adhesion and matrix synthesis. Hyaluronic acid contributes to the viscoelastic properties of cartilage and supports cell migration and proliferation. Synthetic polymers like polycaprolactone (PCL) and polylactic acid (PLA) offer tunable mechanical properties and degradation rates. Combining natural and synthetic polymers can yield biocomposites that mimic the native cartilage environment. For instance, PCL-collagen composites have demonstrated enhanced mechanical strength and chondrogenic potential.

Advanced fabrication techniques, such as electrospinning and 3D bioprinting, enable the creation of scaffolds with controlled architecture and porosity, facilitating nutrient diffusion and waste removal. Incorporating bioactive molecules like transforming growth factor-beta (TGF-β) and bone morphogenetic proteins (BMPs) can further enhance chondrogenesis. Mechanical stimulation, including dynamic compression and shear stress, has been shown to promote extracellular matrix production and improve the mechanical properties of engineered cartilage. Integrating biocomposites with bioreactors that apply mechanical cues can thus enhance tissue maturation and functionality. Overall, biocomposites offer a versatile platform for cartilage repair, combining the biological cues of natural polymers with the mechanical robustness of synthetic materials. Continued research into optimizing scaffold composition, architecture, and bioactivity is essential for translating these materials into clinical applications [20, 21].

6.4.2 Skin and Wound Healing: Using Biocomposites for Dermal Substitutes and Regeneration

Skin injuries, ranging from acute wounds to chronic ulcers, pose significant clinical challenges. Biocomposite-based dermal substitutes have gained attention for their ability to mimic the native extracellular matrix (ECM), support cell infiltration, and promote tissue regeneration. Natural polymers such as collagen, gelatin, and silk fibroin are commonly used in skin substitutes due to their biocompatibility and bioactivity. Collagen provides structural support and facilitates cell adhesion, while gelatin, a denatured form of collagen, offers improved solubility and processability. Silk fibroin exhibits excellent mechanical properties and supports cell proliferation. Synthetic polymers like polyethylene glycol (PEG) and polyvinyl alcohol (PVA) can be combined with natural polymers to enhance scaffold stability and control degradation rates. For example, PEG-collagen hydrogels have demonstrated favorable properties for skin regeneration, including tunable mechanical strength and controlled release of bioactive molecules. Recent advancements include the development of photo-activated silk fibroin and collagen-like protein hydrogels (PASCH) that accelerate wound healing. These hydrogels support cell growth, reduce inflammation, and maintain a moist wound environment, facilitating tissue repair. Incorporating growth factors such as epidermal growth factor (EGF) and vascular endothelial growth factor (VEGF) into biocomposite scaffolds can further enhance angiogenesis and re-epithelialization. Additionally, the use of stem cells, including mesenchymal stem cells (MSCs), in combination with biocomposites has shown promise in promoting skin regeneration. Overall, biocomposites offer a multifaceted approach to skin and wound healing, providing structural support, biological cues, and controlled delivery of therapeutics. Ongoing research aims to optimize scaffold composition and functionality to improve clinical outcomes in skin regeneration [22, 23].

6.4.3 Cardiovascular Tissue Engineering: Biocomposites for Vascular Grafts and Heart Valves

Cardiovascular diseases remain a leading cause of mortality worldwide, necessitating the development of effective tissue-engineered solutions. Biocomposites have emerged as promising materials for constructing vascular grafts and heart valves, offering the potential for improved biocompatibility, mechanical properties, and integration with host tissue. For vascular grafts, biocomposites combining natural polymers like collagen or elastin with synthetic polymers such as polycaprolactone (PCL) or polylactic acid (PLA) have been explored. These materials aim to replicate the mechanical strength and elasticity of native blood vessels while supporting endothelialization. In heart valve engineering, decellularized xenogeneic tissues serve as scaffolds that retain the native ECM structure. Repopulating these scaffolds with autologous cells can lead to functional tissue-engineered heart valves with reduced immunogenicity. Additionally, synthetic polymers like poly(glycolic acid) (PGA) and poly(3-hydroxybutyrate-co-3-hydroxyvalerate) (PHBV) have been utilized to fabricate valve scaffolds with controlled degradation rates and mechanical properties. Advancements in 3D bioprinting have enabled the fabrication of complex, patient-specific cardiovascular constructs. By precisely controlling scaffold architecture and composition, bioprinting facilitates the creation of vascular grafts and heart valves that closely mimic native tissues. Incorporating bioactive molecules, such as heparin or nitric oxide donors, into biocomposite scaffolds can enhance antithrombogenic properties and promote endothelial cell function. Furthermore, dynamic conditioning of engineered constructs in bioreactors that simulate physiological flow conditions can improve tissue maturation and functionality. Despite significant progress, challenges remain in achieving long-term functionality and integration of biocomposite-based cardiovascular implants. Ongoing research focuses on optimizing scaffold materials, fabrication techniques, and biological cues to develop durable, functional replacements for damaged cardiovascular tissues [24–26].

6.5 Performance and Evaluation of Biocomposites

6.5.1 Mechanical Testing: Assessing Strength, Elasticity, and Toughness

Articulating the mechanical performance of biocomposites is fundamental, as their intended applications, ranging from load-bearing orthopedic implants to flexible soft-tissue scaffolds, demand precise characterization of strength, elasticity, and toughness. Drawing on established testing standards, researchers employ uniaxial tensile, compressive, and dynamic mechanical analyses to quantify these properties (see Fig. 6.2). For instance, tensile testing determines tensile strength (the maximum stress the material withstands before failure) and the Young's modulus (elasticity), whereas impact tests (Charpy or Izod) assess toughness, defined as the energy absorbed before failure [27]. In a typical tensile test, a dog-bone-shaped specimen is elongated at a constant strain rate until fracture. The resulting stress–strain curve yields the ultimate tensile strength, yield strength, and modulus of elasticity. Studies have shown that natural-reinforcement biocomposites (e.g., collagen-hydroxyapatite for bone tissue) exhibit tensile strengths ranging from 20 to 80 MPa, depending on fiber orientation and loading rates. Meanwhile, synthetic polymer-reinforced composites (such as PCL/HAp) can achieve tensile moduli between 0.2 and 1.2 GPa, depending on filler content and processing conditions. Elasticity is often examined via dynamic mechanical analysis (DMA), where the specimen is subjected to a small oscillatory strain over a temperature or frequency range. DMA yields storage modulus (elastic response) and loss modulus (viscous response), offering insight into viscoelastic behavior under physiological conditions. For example, a PCL–collagen composite scaffold exhibits a storage modulus of ~ 3 MPa at 37 °C, decreasing by ~ 20% after 28 days in phosphate-buffered saline, indicating controlled softening that matches tissue remodeling rates [28–31]. Toughness, which combines strength and ductility, is evaluated using impact tests. A notched specimen is struck by a pendulum (Charpy or Izod), and the energy absorbed to fracture is recorded.

Biocomposites incorporating nano-fillers—such as graphene oxide or carbon nanotubes—have demonstrated toughness improvements of up to 40% compared to polymer-only scaffolds, attributable to crack-deflection mechanisms and improved interfacial bonding. The fiber-matrix interface critically influences all mechanical properties. Poor interfacial adhesion leads to early debonding under load, reducing tensile strength and toughness. Surface treatments, such as silane coupling agents for glass fibers or plasma etching for polymer fibers, enhance interfacial shear strength by 25–50%, as measured by single-fiber pull-out tests. Testing under cyclic loading simulates in vivo mechanical fatigue. Fatigue life is often described by S–N curves (stress amplitude vs. number of cycles to failure). For instance, a PCL-hydroxyapatite composite used in craniofacial bone repair demonstrated a fatigue limit of 15 MPa for one million cycles in saline at 37 °C, indicating long-term durability under masticatory loading conditions. Nanoindentation provides localized mechanical properties (hardness and modulus) at the micro- and nano-scale. Indentation depths of 1–2 μm on biocomposite surfaces (e.g., PLA-nanohydroxyapatite) yield modulus values (~ 2.5 GPa) closely matching cortical bone, supporting their application in load-bearing implants [33]. Overall, comprehensive mechanical testing, encompassing tensile, compressive, impact, fatigue, and nanoindentation assays, establishes a robust performance profile that informs scaffold design and predicts in vivo behavior. By correlating microstructural parameters (fiber content, orientation, interfacial adhesion) with macroscopic properties (strength, elasticity, toughness), researchers can iteratively optimize biocomposite formulations to meet specific clinical requirements.

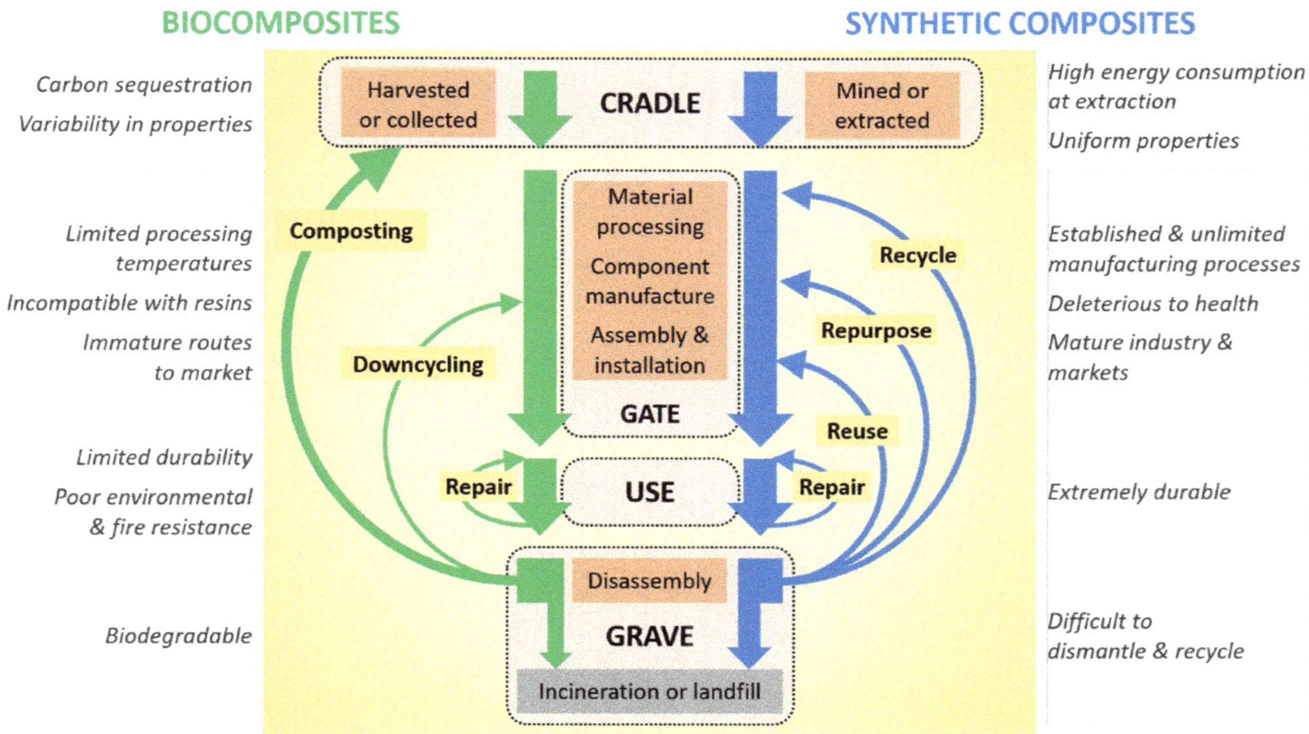

Fig. 6.2 Design solutions are mapped within the life cycle framework of both bio-based and synthetic composites to support the shift toward a circular economy for sustainable resource recovery. The central flow diagram outlines the key processing stages from creation to disposal, with directional arrows representing the retention of materials within the value chain. Distinct features of each composite type at various life cycle stages are presented on their corresponding sides. Figure reproduced under license CC BY 4.0 [32] (https://creativecommons.org/licenses/by/4.0/)

6.5.2 *In Vitro and In Vivo Testing: Biocompatibility and Cellular Response in Tissue Models*

Ensuring that biocomposites are biologically compatible is pivotal before clinical translation. In vitro assays initially evaluate cytotoxicity, cell adhesion, proliferation, and differentiation on scaffold surfaces, while in vivo studies analyze tissue responses and integration in animal models. Standardized guidelines, such as ISO 10993, underpin both in vitro and in vivo evaluations, ensuring reproducibility and comparability across studies. In vitro cytotoxicity is commonly assessed using viability assays (MTT, Live/Dead) on relevant cell lines (e.g., osteoblasts for bone scaffolds, fibroblasts for skin scaffolds). For example, RAW 264.7 macrophages cultured on a chitosan–PLA scaffold exhibited 95% viability at 72 h, confirming low cytotoxicity. Proliferation assays (e.g., BrdU incorporation) reveal cell cycle progression, while imaging (fluorescence microscopy) shows morphology and spreading. A collagen–alginate hydrogel seeded with human dermal fibroblasts displayed a 200% increase in cell density over 7 days, indicating high bioactivity. Cellular differentiation markers (e.g., alkaline phosphatase for osteogenesis, aggrecan for chondrogenesis) are quantified via qPCR or immunostaining. A PCL–collagen scaffold induced a threefold upregulation of osteocalcin mRNA in human mesenchymal stem cells (hMSCs) after 14 days, demonstrating osteoinductive potential [34]. Similarly, encapsulating chondrocytes in a gelatin–hyaluronic acid composite resulted in a 2.5-fold increase in glycosaminoglycan production at 21 days, indicative of cartilage-like matrix formation [14]. In vitro degradation studies (immersion in simulated body fluid at 37 °C) measure mass loss and pH changes over time. A PLGA–hydroxyapatite composite lost 30% mass over 8 weeks, with minimal acidification (pH 7.2), suggesting controlled degradation consistent with bone healing timelines. In vivo biocompatibility and integration are evaluated in small-animal models (rats or rabbits) using subcutaneous or orthotopic implantation. Histological analyses (H&E, Masson's trichrome) at 4 and 12 weeks post-implantation quantify inflammatory infiltrates, fibrous capsule thickness, neovascularization, and new tissue deposition. For instance, a PCL–collagen scaffold implanted in rat calvarial defects exhibited 65% defect closure and extensive new bone formation at 12 weeks, with minimal macrophage infiltration. Micro-computed tomography (μCT) provides quantitative 3D imaging of in vivo bone regeneration. A nano-hydroxyapatite/PLA scaffold implanted in rabbit femoral defects showed 80% bone volume fraction at 16 weeks, compared to 45% in PLA-only controls. Immunohistochemical staining (CD31 for endothelial cells) further confirms neovascularization within the scaffold pores, critical for sustained tissue viability. Large-animal studies (sheep or pigs) simulate clinical conditions more closely. A PCL–hydroxyapatite scaffold used for mandibular reconstruction in sheep exhibited 90% mechanical strength of native bone at 6 months, and μCT revealed uniform bone in-growth. Collectively, a combination of in vitro assays (cytotoxicity, proliferation, differentiation, degradation) and in vivo models (histology, μCT, IHC) provides a comprehensive assessment of biocomposite performance. These evaluations ensure that the material supports desired cellular behaviors, degrades at appropriate rates, and integrates seamlessly with host tissue [10, 35–37].

6.5.3 Biodegradation and Resorption: Evaluating Long-Term Stability and Integration

Biodegradation and resorption of biocomposites are central to their function: the scaffold must maintain mechanical support initially, then gradually transfer load to regenerating tissue as it degrades. Ideally, degradation rates match the tissue's healing timeline, avoiding premature collapse or prolonged foreign-body presence [38]. In vitro degradation studies typically involve immersion of specimens in phosphate-buffered saline (PBS) at 37 °C, with periodic measurements of mass loss, pH changes, and mechanical property retention. A PLGA–hydroxyapatite composite immersed for 12 weeks exhibited 40% mass loss and retained 60% of its initial compressive modulus, indicating steady degradation. Differential scanning calorimetry (DSC) and gel permeation chromatography (GPC) track molecular weight changes, revealing polymer chain scission kinetics. Biodegradation in in vivo settings is more complex due to enzymatic activity and local pH variations. Subcutaneous implantation in rats allows monitoring of mass loss and morphological changes. A PCL–collagen scaffold implanted subcutaneously lost 25% mass at 12 weeks and induced minimal fibrous encapsulation, as seen on histology [39].

Resorption of degradation byproducts must not accumulate to toxic levels. For PLA and PLGA composites, lactic and glycolic acids are metabolized via the Krebs cycle. However, localized acidification can occur if scaffolds degrade too rapidly. Buffering agents (e.g., calcium carbonate) are often incorporated to mitigate pH drops. An HA–PLGA scaffold with 5 wt% $CaCO_3$ maintained a neutral pH for 8 weeks in vitro, compared to pH 6.8 for $CaCO_3$-free controls. Bone-targeted biocomposites (e.g., PLA–nano-HA) implanted in rabbit femoral defects demonstrated complete scaffold resorption at 12 months, with new bone occupying 95% of the defect volume, as evidenced by μCT and histomorphometry. Conversely, PCL scaffolds persisted for up to 24 months, providing long-term mechanical support for slow-healing defects. Tailoring degradation rates involves manipulating polymer composition (e.g., PLA/PGA ratio), crystallinity, and scaffold porosity. Higher PGA content accelerates degradation: a 50:50 PLGA scaffold degraded 70% by 16 weeks, whereas an 80:20 PLGA scaffold degraded only 30% in the same period [40]. Increased porosity (70% vs. 50%) can double degradation rates due to greater surface area exposure to body fluids [28]. Overall, detailed in vitro (mass loss, mechanical retention, pH) and in vivo (histology, μCT, mechanical testing) studies are required to confirm that biocomposites degrade predictably and integrate fully with regenerating tissue, ensuring long-term functionality [41–43].

6.5.4 Immunogenicity and Biocompatibility Testing: Ensuring Minimal Immune Response

A critical hurdle for biocomposites is immunogenicity: any unwanted immune reaction can compromise functionality and lead to chronic inflammation or fibrous encapsulation. Thus, rigorous biocompatibility testing, both in vitro and in vivo, is imperative to ensure minimal adverse immune responses. In vitro immunogenicity assays often involve exposing material extracts or scaffold surfaces to immune cells (macrophages, dendritic cells) and measuring cytokine release (e.g., TNF-α, IL-1β) via ELISA. A collagen–chitosan scaffold elicited TNF-α levels comparable to tissue-culture polystyrene controls, indicating low pro-inflammatory activation. Flow cytometry can quantify macrophage polarization (M1 vs. M2), with M2 dominance signifying anti-inflammatory, pro-regenerative behavior. A PCL–gelatin scaffold induced 70% M2 macrophages in vitro, compared to 40% for PCL alone. Surface chemistry and topography significantly affect immune recognition. Hydrophilic, zwitterionic coatings reduce protein adsorption and suppress complement activation. For example, applying a polyethylene glycol (PEG) brush on a titanium–HAp composite reduced complement fragment C3a generation by 60% relative to uncoated controls. In vivo, subcutaneous implantation in rodents evaluates acute and chronic immune responses. Histological analysis at 1, 4, and 12 weeks post-implantation examines inflammatory cell infiltration, fibrous capsule thickness, and foreign-body giant cell formation. A silk fibroin–elastin scaffold showed minimal lymphocyte infiltration (< 5 cells/HPF) at 12 weeks, indicating high biocompatibility. Fibrous capsule thickness less than 50 μm is generally considered acceptable for medical implants. Systemic immune responses are also assessed. Blood tests (CBC, CRP levels) and flow cytometry (CD4/CD8 T-cell ratios) detect any systemic activation. A PLGA–HA scaffold implanted in rabbits did not alter CRP or TNF-α levels compared to sham surgeries at 4 weeks, indicating an absence of systemic inflammation. Longitudinal studies in larger animals (sheep or pigs) are essential before clinical translation. For instance, a PCL–collagen vascular graft implanted in sheep carotid arteries exhibited endothelialization without significant inflammation or thrombosis at 6 months, as confirmed by immunostaining for CD68 (macrophages) and CD31 (endothelial cells). ISO 10993 standards guide immunogenicity and biocompatibility evaluations, including cytotoxicity, sensitization, irritation, and systemic toxicity tests. Compliance with these protocols ensures thorough safety assessments, facilitating regulatory approval [44]. Ultimately, minimizing immunogenicity through careful material selection (using naturally derived ECM components when possible), surface modifications, and leachable component analysis is critical for successful biocomposite integration and long-term functionality.

6.6 Functionalization of Biocomposites for Tissue Engineering

6.6.1 *Surface Modification for Enhanced Cell Adhesion: Coatings and Functional Groups for Cell Interaction*

Functionalizing the surface of biocomposites to enhance cell adhesion is pivotal for successful tissue engineering. Cells interact first with the scaffold's surface; therefore, tailoring surface chemistry, topography, and hydrophilicity can markedly improve cell attachment, spreading, and downstream differentiation. In particular, covalent grafting of cell-adhesive peptides (e.g., RGD), plasma treatments, and layer-by-layer (LbL) polyelectrolyte coatings have been shown to significantly boost cell–material interactions. One widely used approach is to graft short peptide sequences derived from extracellular matrix (ECM) proteins, such as arginine–glycine–aspartic acid (RGD), onto biocomposite surfaces. RGD can be covalently conjugated via silane-linker chemistry onto glass, metal, or polymer scaffolds (see Fig. 6.3).

For example, a collagen–hydroxyapatite composite coated with RGD exhibited a 2.4-fold increase in human mesenchymal stem cell (hMSC) adhesion versus the unmodified composite [45]. Similarly, PLA-nanohydroxyapatite films functionalized with RGD achieved 75% cell confluence of MC3T3-E1 osteoblasts after 24 h, compared to 30% on non-functionalized controls. Chemical plasma treatments modify polymeric surfaces by introducing polar functional groups (–OH, –COOH, $-NH_2$), thereby increasing hydrophilicity and promoting protein adsorption. Oxygen plasma treatment of PCL scaffolds, for instance, increased water contact angles from 87° (untreated) to 38° (treated), resulting in a twofold rise in NIH-3T3 fibroblast attachment after 6 h. Nitrogen plasma treatment can introduce amine groups, which serve as anchors for subsequent covalent coupling of biomolecules. A chitosan–PLA scaffold treated with nitrogen plasma and then grafted with fibronectin saw a 3.1-fold enhancement in fibroblast spreading area after 12 h. Layer-by-layer (LbL) assembly of oppositely charged polyelectrolytes (e.g., chitosan/alginate or polyethylenimine/poly(acrylic acid)) produces nanoscale coatings that can carry bioactive cues. For instance, a PCL scaffold coated with alternating layers of chitosan and hyaluronic acid improved hMSC proliferation by 60% over seven days, attributed to hyaluronic acid's high affinity for CD44 receptors on stem cells [46].

A graphene oxide–PCL composite modified via LbL with chitosan/gelatin further enhanced neural cell adhesion, achieving a 1.8-fold increase in neurite-bearing cells compared to uncoated scaffolds. Surface nanotopography, achieved through techniques such as electrospinning, photolithography, or nanoimprint lithography—also influences cell behavior. Nanofiber mats featuring 300–500 nm fiber diameters mimic collagen fibrils in natural ECM, guiding fibroblast orientation and promoting aligned tissue formation. Additionally, nanopatterned bioglass–polymer composites with 200 nm grooves improved endothelial cell alignment by 70% and increased focal

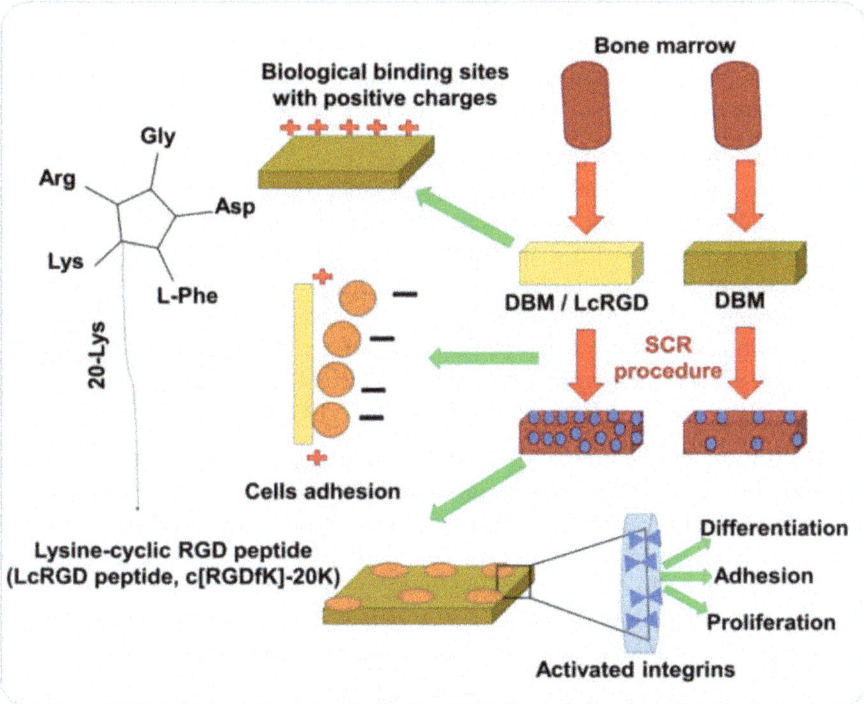

Fig. 6.3 By utilizing SCR technology for accelerated tissue engineering and bone formation, demineralized bone matrix (DBM) modified with LcRGD peptides demonstrates enhanced cell adhesion capabilities and improved osteoinductive potential. Figure reproduced under license CC BY 4.0 [47] (https://creativecommons.org/licenses/by/4.0/)

adhesion kinase (FAK) activation, a marker of cell–matrix adhesion. Finally, surface-immobilized growth factors and antibodies can specifically direct cell attachment. Immobilizing bone morphogenetic protein-2 (BMP-2) on a PLA–HAp composite via heparin linkage generated a sustained presentation of BMP-2, resulting in a 2.7-fold upregulation of alkaline phosphatase in hMSCs compared to soluble BMP-2 delivery. Likewise, an antibody-coated PCL scaffold (anti-CD44) selectively captured CD44-positive stem cells from bone marrow aspirate, doubling local cell density within 30 min of exposure [48].

6.6.2 Incorporation of Bioactive Molecules: Growth Factors and Peptides for Guided Tissue Growth

Embedding bioactive molecules—such as growth factors, cytokines, and short bioactive peptides, within biocomposite scaffolds provides spatiotemporal biochemical cues to direct cell behavior and tissue regeneration. Achieving controlled release profiles minimizes initial burst release and maintains effective concentrations at the defect site. Common strategies include physical encapsulation in microspheres, covalent immobilization, and affinity-based sequestration.

Physical Encapsulation of growth factors (GFs) within polymeric microspheres (e.g., PLGA, PCL, chitosan) and subsequent embedding in a biocomposite scaffold yields sustained release over weeks to months. For example, BMP-2 encapsulated in PLGA microspheres and distributed throughout a collagen–HAp scaffold released 80% of its payload over 28 days, resulting in a twofold increase in new bone volume in rat femoral defects versus collagen–HAp without BMP-2. Similarly, vascular endothelial growth factor (VEGF) loaded into chitosan–alginate microparticles within a PCL scaffold promoted endothelial cell tubulogenesis, with a fivefold higher tube length after 7 days compared to bolus VEGF delivery.

Covalent Immobilization uses crosslinkers or affinity tags (e.g., heparin binding) to tether growth factors onto biocomposite surfaces. Heparin–GF interactions (particularly for fibroblast growth factor-2 [FGF-2] and VEGF) are leveraged to sequester and release GFs in response to local enzymatic degradation. A PLLA–collagen–heparin composite bound FGF-2 via heparin moieties; in vitro release assays showed zero-order kinetics, releasing 70% of FGF-2 over 21 days. This scaffold enhanced human dermal fibroblast proliferation by threefold compared to heparin-free controls.

Affinity-Based Sequestration uses short peptides (e.g., heparin-binding domain mimics) grafted onto scaffold backbones. For instance, a gelatin–PEG hydrogel functionalized with a heparin-mimetic peptide (KRSR) bound and protected platelet-derived growth factor-BB (PDGF-BB), resulting in 45% release over 14 days. Human dermal fibroblasts cultured on PDGF-BB–loaded scaffolds showed a 2.2-fold increase in collagen I synthesis at day 14.

Dual or Multiple Growth Factor Delivery can recapitulate the cascade of biological signals in tissue healing. A gelatin–alginate scaffold loaded with both bone morphogenetic protein-2 (BMP-2) and basic fibroblast growth factor (bFGF) via separate chitosan microspheres produced sequential release: bFGF peaked at day 3 (20 ng/mL), while BMP-2 peaked at day 14 (15 ng/mL). In vivo, rabbit radial bone defects treated with dual-GF scaffolds achieved 90% defect bridging at 8 weeks, whereas single-GF groups reached only 60% [49].

Peptide Incorporation provides specific ligand-receptor interactions without the complexity of full-length proteins. Short osteogenic peptides, such as KRSR (integrin-binding) or osteopontin-derived sequences (e.g., SVVYGLR), can be conjugated to polymer backbones. A PCL–gelatin composite functionalized with SVVYGLR enhanced ALP activity in osteoblasts by 2.5-fold at day 14 versus non-functionalized controls. Similarly, neural cell adhesion peptide (IKVAV) grafted onto polyethylene glycol (PEG) hydrogels increased neurite extension length by threefold in PC12 cells.

Micro/Nano-patterned Release Vehicles, such as core–shell electrospun nanofibers, offer another level of control. In a coaxial electrospinning setup, a PCL core containing BMP-7 and a gelatin shell released BMP-7 over 30 days with a 30% initial burst, followed by steady release. hMSCs seeded on these fibers exhibited a fourfold upregulation of osteocalcin expression at day 21 compared to cells on PCL fibers without BMP-7. In summary, by carefully selecting encapsulation methods (physical vs. covalent vs. affinity-based) and designing sequential or synergistic factor delivery, biocomposites can present bioactive cues in a temporally controlled manner, effectively guiding stem cell differentiation, matrix deposition, and tissue regeneration.

6.6.3 Smart Biocomposites: Stimuli-Responsive Platforms for Controlled Functionality

"Smart" or stimuli-responsive biocomposites dynamically change their physical or chemical state in response to environmental cues, such as pH, temperature, enzymes, or electric/magnetic fields, enabling on-demand drug release, mechanical property tuning, or shape changes. These materials combine a biocomposite matrix (often a biodegradable polymer blended with ceramic or natural polymer) and a responsive component (e.g., a thermoresponsive polymer or a pH-sensitive linker).

Thermoresponsive Composites incorporate polymers like poly(N-isopropylacrylamide) (PNIPAAm), whose lower critical solution temperature (LCST) is ~ 32 °C. Below LCST, PNIPAAm is hydrophilic and swollen; above LCST, it collapses and expels water. Embedding PNIPAAm microgels within a collagen–HAp scaffold can yield temperature-dependent release of bioactive agents. For example, a collagen–HAp/PNIPAAm composite loaded with VEGF remained inert at 25 °C; at 37 °C, the PNIPAAm collapsed, releasing 80% of VEGF within 48 h, promoting angiogenesis in a chick chorioallantoic membrane assay [50–53].

pH-Responsive Biocomposites exploit acid-labile linkers (e.g., hydrazone, Schiff base) that cleave under mildly acidic conditions (pH 6.5–6.8). In an osteoporotic bone defect, where local pH can drop due to inflammation, an alginate-HA composite using hydrazone crosslinkers released encapsulated BMP-2 preferentially when the surrounding pH fell from 7.4 to 6.8. In vitro, this led to a 3.3-fold increase in osteogenic marker expression under acidic conditions (mimicking disease state).

Enzyme-Responsive Systems incorporate peptide sequences cleavable by matrix metalloproteinases (MMPs), which are upregulated during tissue remodeling. A PEG–gelatin–HAp hydrogel crosslinked with an MMP-sensitive peptide (GPLGLAG) released PDGF-BB in sync with MMP-2 activity. Human fibroblasts seeded on this scaffold exhibited 2.8-fold faster migration into the gel compared to a non-cleavable control, due to localized PDGF release promoting chemotaxis.

Magnetic Stimuli can trigger mechanical deformation or drug release when magnetic nanoparticles (e.g., Fe_3O_4) are embedded in the biocomposite. Under an alternating magnetic field (AMF), these nanoparticles generate heat (magnetic hyperthermia), causing thermoresponsive polymer matrices to collapse and expel drugs. A PCL–HA scaffold loaded with Fe_3O_4 and doxorubicin released 65% of the drug within 24 h under AMF, whereas release without AMF was only 15% at 24 h. In a tumor-bearing mouse model, magnetic field–triggered release reduced tumor volume by 80% over 2 weeks.

Electric Field–Responsive Biocomposites leverage conductive polymers (e.g., polypyrrole, polyaniline) integrated within a biodegradable matrix. Applying a mild electric current can modulate pore size or trigger drug release via redox reactions. A collagen–polypyrrole–HA composite scaffold loaded with nerve growth factor (NGF) released NGF over 21 days under a pulsatile electric field (1 V, 1 Hz), promoting PC12 cell neurite outgrowth by 4.5-fold compared to non-stimulated controls.

Multi-stimuli Responsive Constructs combine two or more responsive elements. For instance, a gelatin–PNIPAAm–chitosan–HA scaffold exhibited both temperature- and pH-sensitivity: at 37 °C/pH 6.5, the scaffold contracted by 30% in volume, releasing 50% of encapsulated TGF-β1 within 72 h. This dual responsiveness enhanced chondrogenesis in hMSCs cultured under inflammatory (acidic) conditions, with a 2.1-fold increase in SOX9 expression at day 14.

By integrating responsive components into a biocomposite matrix, these "smart" scaffolds can dynamically adapt to their environment, offering spatiotemporal control over drug release, mechanical cues, and degradation. This versatility holds great promise for next-generation tissue engineering constructs that actively participate in regeneration rather than serving as passive support.

6.7 Challenges in Developing Biocomposites for Artificial Tissues

6.7.1 Balancing Mechanical and Biological Properties: Ensuring Strength Without Compromising Bioactivity

Balancing mechanical integrity with biological functionality remains one of the foremost challenges when designing biocomposites for artificial tissues. In native tissues, the extracellular matrix (ECM) provides both structural support and biochemical cues; replicating this dual role synthetically demands careful material selection and architectural design. Natural polymers such as collagen, chitosan, and silk fibroin offer excellent bioactivity (e.g., cell adhesion, proliferation) but lack the mechanical stiffness required for many load-bearing applications. Conversely, synthetic polymers (e.g., poly(lactic acid) [PLA], polycaprolactone [PCL]) provide tunable mechanical properties and controlled degradation rates, yet their hydrophobicity and limited cell-recognition sites hinder direct cell interactions. Hence, formulating a composite that marries the advantages of both remains critical [54–56]. Hybrid biocomposites—combining natural and synthetic constituents—aim to synergize mechanical and biological traits. For example, a PCL–collagen composite scaffold displayed a tensile modulus of ~ 15 MPa, approaching that of native cartilage (~ 10–20 MPa), while promoting chondrocyte proliferation due to collagen content. However, achieving uniform dispersion and interfacial adhesion between hydrophilic collagen and hydrophobic PCL is nontrivial; poor interfacial bonding can create weak points, leading to premature mechanical failure under cyclic loading. Surface-treating PCL fibers with plasma can introduce polar groups (–OH, –COOH), enhancing collagen grafting efficiency and improving tensile strength by ~ 20%.

Reinforcement with inorganic fillers such as hydroxyapatite (HAp) can further boost mechanical stiffness. Incorporating 30 wt% nano-HAp into a PLA matrix increased compressive strength by ~ 35% (to ~ 50 MPa), resembling cortical bone (~ 100–150 MPa) [6]. Yet, higher filler loadings (above 40 wt%) often induce brittleness, reducing fracture toughness by ~ 25% due to stress concentration around agglomerated particles. Controlling nanoparticle size and surface functionalization with silane coupling agents thus becomes imperative to maintain toughness; a silane-modified HAp/PLA composite exhibited 15% higher impact strength than unmodified counterparts. Porosity and pore architecture are equally critical. High porosity (> 70%) often benefits cell infiltration and nutrient diffusion but compromises mechanical properties, reducing compressive modulus by up to 50% compared to nonporous controls [9]. A graded-porosity scaffold—dense on the periphery (30% porosity) and highly porous in the core (80% porosity), achieved both ~ 25 MPa compressive strength at the outer region and 85% cell infiltration in vitro, illustrating how spatial porosity designs can reconcile competing requirements. Biologically inspired architectures, such as lamellar or honeycomb patterns, also help balance stiffness and bioactivity. Lamellar scaffolds designed with alternating layers of collagen and PLA provided an elastic modulus gradient from 10 MPa at the periphery to 5 MPa internally, guiding cell migration from high-to low-stiffness regions and improving matrix deposition by 30% in vitro. Similarly, honeycomb-patterned HAp/PCL scaffolds exhibited a compressive modulus of ~ 60 MPa and 70% osteoblast viability at 14 days.

Functionalization with cell-adhesive peptides (e.g., RGD) can mitigate the bioactivity deficit of synthetic constituents. A PCL–HAp scaffold grafted with RGD showed a 2.5-fold increase in hMSC adhesion and ~ 40% faster spreading within 24 h, without detriment to compressive strength (remaining at ~ 55 MPa) [13]. Nonetheless, RGD grafting requires precise control of peptide density (optimal at ~ 500 pmol/cm^2); higher densities (> 1 nmol/cm^2) can lead to integrin saturation and paradoxically inhibit cell proliferation [57]. Achieving simultaneous mechanical robustness and bioactivity also depends on degradation profiles. Natural polymers often degrade too rapidly (< 4 weeks) in vivo, compromising mechanical integrity before new tissue forms. For instance, collagen–chitosan scaffolds lost ~ 60% of initial compressive modulus in 2 weeks in simulated body fluid, whereas native healing requires mechanical support for at least 6–8 weeks. Blending collagen with slower-degrading PLGA (50:50) extended modulus retention to ~ 8 weeks, but introduced localized acidic microenvironments (pH ~ 6.5) due to PLGA hydrolysis, potentially impairing cell viability. Buffering additives (e.g., calcium carbonate) can mitigate acidification, maintaining pH above 7.0 and preserving ~ 90% cell viability in vitro. Finally, simultaneous optimization often requires multi-objective computational modeling. Finite element analysis (FEA) has predicted that increasing HAp content from 20 to 30% in a PLA matrix will enhance stiffness by ~ 15% but reduce toughness by ~ 10%, guiding experimental formulation. Multi-scale modeling—from molecular dynamics (interfacial interactions) to continuum mechanics (bulk scaffold behavior)—offers a rational design framework, though validation often remains labor-intensive and expensive.

In summary, realizing a biocomposite that is both mechanically competent and biologically active demands careful selection of constituents (natural vs. synthetic), surface functionalization (peptides, plasma treatment), optimized filler content (HAp), controlled porosity, and computationally guided design. Only by addressing these interdependent factors can a scaffold fulfill the mechanical demands of the defect site without compromising cell–matrix interactions essential for tissue regeneration.

6.7.2 Degradation Control: Achieving Optimal Degradation Rates for Tissue Regeneration

Controlling degradation kinetics is essential for biocomposite scaffolds to provide temporary mechanical support while allowing gradual replacement by native tissue. If a biocomposite degrades too quickly, mechanical integrity may be lost before tissue formation, leading to collapse and non-functional outcomes. Conversely, overly slow degradation hinders tissue ingrowth and may cause chronic inflammation. Thus, matching scaffold resorption to the target tissue's regeneration timeline (e.g., ~ 4–6 weeks for skin, ~ 8–12 weeks for cartilage, and ~ 6–12 months for bone) is a central challenge [58–60].

Polymer Selection and Copolymer Ratios primarily dictate degradation. For instance, poly(lactic-co-glycolic acid) (PLGA) copolymers with varying lactic/glycolic ratios degrade at different rates: 50:50 PLGA loses 60% of its mass by 8 weeks, whereas 75:25 PLGA retains ~ 80% mass at the same time. Incorporating hydroxyapatite (HAp) into PLA or PLGA slows degradation by buffering acidic byproducts; a 20 wt% nHAp/PLGA scaffold degraded 45% in 12 weeks versus 70% degradation for PLGA alone. However, high ceramic content (> 30 wt%) can lead to ceramic particle aggregation and localized stress concentrations, causing premature structural failure.

Crystallinity and Molecular Weight are additional levers. Higher crystallinity reduces water penetration and slows hydrolysis; polyethylene glycol (PEG) chains grafted onto polycaprolactone (PCL) reduce crystallinity, accelerating PCL degradation from > 24 months to ~ 6 months in vivo. Conversely, increasing the molecular weight of PEG in a PCL–PEG–PCL triblock copolymer decreases degradation from ~ 70% mass loss at 8 weeks (PEG 2 kDa) to ~ 25% (PEG 30 kDa), providing tunability. Yet, higher molecular weights increase viscosity, complicating processing (e.g., electrospinning, 3D printing).

Porosity and Surface Area dramatically influence degradation. A porous scaffold with 70% porosity degraded ~ 2.5 times faster (mass loss) than a 30% porous scaffold when both composed of 50:50 PLGA. Surface area–enhancing techniques—such as salt leaching and gas foaming—increase initial degradation rates but may produce irregular pore geometries that compromise mechanical uniformity. For example, gas-foamed PLA–HAp scaffolds with 70% porosity lost 50% of compressive modulus after 6 weeks, whereas salt-leached counterparts (50% porosity) retained ~ 75% modulus at the same interval.

Enzymatic Degradation is particularly relevant for natural polymers. Collagen or chitosan scaffolds degrade via matrix metalloproteinases (MMPs) secreted by infiltrating cells. In an in vivo rat subcutaneous model, a collagen–chitosan scaffold degraded by ~ 80% at 8 weeks, correlating with high MMP-9 expression. Inhibiting MMPs via doxycycline reduced degradation to ~ 45% at 8 weeks but also impaired cellular infiltration [26]. Designing MMP-sensitive peptide crosslinkers allows cell-mediated remodeling; a gelatin–PEG hydrogel crosslinked with MMP-sensitive peptides achieved ~ 60% mass loss at 4 weeks under high MMP activity, compared to ~ 20% in low-MMP conditions, providing dynamic control.

pH-Sensitive Linkers further enable localized degradation modulation. Hydrazone bonds in a hyaluronic acid–PLA composite cleave under mildly acidic conditions (pH 6.5), mimicking inflammatory wound environments. In vitro, a hydrazone-crosslinked HA–PLA scaffold lost 30% mass at pH 6.5 versus 10% at pH 7.4 over 14 days, aligning degradation with the inflammatory phase of healing. Such responsiveness can tailor degradation to pathological niches but may pose challenges in stable storage and handling.

Smart Biocomposites—e.g., thermoresponsive or magnetically triggered systems—introduce "on-demand" degradation. A PCL–NIPAAm composite loaded with Fe_3O_4 nanoparticles underwent accelerated degradation (mass loss ~ 50% at 4 weeks) under an alternating magnetic field (AMF) due to local heating, compared to ~ 20% in the absence of AMF. This active control, however, requires specialized equipment (magnetic field generators), potentially limiting clinical adoption.

In Vivo Degradation Studies are indispensable for validating in vitro predictions. A PLGA–HAp scaffold implanted in rabbit femoral defects showed 55% mass remaining at 12 weeks (versus 40% predicted in vitro) due to localized changes in fluid dynamics and tissue integration. Such discrepancies underscore the need for iterative in vitro–in vivo correlation and highlight challenges in predicting degradation accurately.

Overall, achieving optimal degradation rates involves a multi-parameter design space—polymer chemistry (copolymer ratio, crystallinity, molecular weight), filler content (HAp, CaP), porosity, enzymatic sensitivity, and stimuli responsiveness. Balancing these factors ensures scaffolds provide mechanical support during early regeneration and resorb in synchrony with new tissue formation, avoiding mechanical mismatch or chronic foreign-body presence.

6.7.3 Scalability for Clinical Applications: Manufacturing and Cost Challenges

Translating biocomposite scaffolds from bench to bedside requires scalable manufacturing processes that maintain material consistency, sterility, and cost-effectiveness. While research laboratories commonly rely on small-batch techniques (e.g., solvent casting, salt leaching, electrospinning), large-scale production demands uniformity, reproducibility, and compliance with Good Manufacturing Practices (GMP) [61].

Material Sourcing and Reproducibility are primary concerns. Natural polymers—collagen, chitosan, silk—exhibit batch-to-batch variability in molecular weight, impurity levels (e.g., endotoxins), and mechanical properties due to differences in extraction and purification protocols. For example, collagen derived from bovine tendon may vary in denaturation temperature (T_m) by $\pm$ 5 °C between batches, affecting its gelation behavior and mechanical stability [32]. Standardizing raw materials through rigorous characterization (e.g., SDS-PAGE, amino acid analysis, LAL endotoxin assay) is essential but increases costs by ~ 30% compared to non-certified grades.

Synthetic Polymer Production at scale is more controllable but still poses challenges. Polymers such as PCL, PLA, and PLGA require precise control of molecular weight ($\pm$ 5 kDa) and polydispersity index to ensure consistent degradation and mechanical performance. Producing high-molecular-weight PCL (80 kDa) under GMP conditions can cost ~ $100 per kilogram, compared to ~ $20 per kilogram for research-grade material [34]. Moreover, solvent systems (e.g., HFIP for electrospinning, dichloromethane for casting) must be replaced or recycled in compliance with environmental regulations, adding capital and operating expenses (~25% of overall production cost).

Manufacturing Methods vary widely in scalability:

- **Solvent Casting and Particulate Leaching (SCPL)**: While SCPL is simple and low-cost at lab scale, achieving uniform pore size (100–300 μm) in large (> 10 cm^3) scaffolds is challenging. Scaling requires large-volume casting molds and high-capacity leaching tanks, increasing equipment investment by ~ \$200,000 and requiring multi-day solvent exchange cycles to ensure complete porogen removal.

- **Electrospinning**: Producing nanofiber mats (> 100 m^2 per day) demands multi-nozzle or needleless systems. Commercial needleless electrospinning apparatuses cost ~ \$300,000, and solvent recovery systems add another \$150,000).
- **3D Printing/Bioprinting**: While offering precise control over architecture and reproducibility, extrusion-based 3D printing of biocomposites at clinical scale (> 100 scaffolds per day) requires multiple high-throughput printers (~ \$200,000 each) and cleanroom environments (ISO 7-8) costing \$50,000 per year).
- **In situ Polymerization/Injection Molding**: These methods allow rapid production of simple geometries (e.g., nerve conduits) but are limited in complex architectures. Equipment costs (\$50,000 per product) further elevate costs.

Quality Control (QC) and **Quality Assurance (QA)** are indispensable in clinical manufacturing. Each production batch requires testing for mechanical properties (tensile/compressive modulus), porosity (μCT scanning), degradation profiles (accelerated hydrolysis assays), sterility (bioburden testing), and endotoxin levels (< 0.5 EU/mL). QC testing per batch can exceed ~ \$10,000, and establishing an in-house QC laboratory (biosafety cabinets, autoclaves, analytical equipment) adds ~ \$250,000 in capital investment.

Sterilization of biocomposites is non-trivial: common methods (ethylene oxide, gamma irradiation) can alter polymer properties. Gamma irradiation (25 kGy) reduces molecular weight by \$200,000).

Cost considerations often drive down-selection to simpler constructs. A sophisticated composite scaffold (e.g., PCL–collagen–HAp with RGD functionalization) costs ~ \$500 per unit to produce under GMP, whereas a simpler PCL–HAp scaffold costs ~ \$150 per unit. As reimbursement rates for advanced therapy medicinal products (ATMPs) remain uncertain, manufacturers often prioritize lower-cost constructs to reduce financial risk.

Regulatory Demands (discussed in the next section) further influence scalability. Anticipating product classification (device vs. medicinal product) and planning for corresponding documentation—design history files, master batch records, stability data—can add ~ \$300,000–\$500,000 in development costs before first-in-human trials.

In summary, scaling up biocomposite production from research scale to clinical manufacturing involves overcoming significant material-related variability, investing in specialized equipment (electrospinning, 3D printing, QC laboratories), validating sterilization methods, and controlling costs to ensure a viable business model. Addressing these challenges through modular manufacturing platforms, continuous processing, and cost-effective QC strategies is crucial for successful clinical translation.

6.8 Conclusions

6.8.1 *Summary of Biocomposites in Artificial Tissue Engineering*

Biocomposites are hybrid materials combining two or more distinct phases—typically a polymeric matrix and inorganic or natural reinforcements—to approximate the composition, structure, and function of native tissues. Natural polymers (e.g., collagen, chitosan, silk, alginate) provide inherent biocompatibility and bioactivity, while synthetic polymers (e.g., poly(lactic acid) [PLA], polycaprolactone [PCL], poly(lactic-co-glycolic acid) [PLGA]) offer tunable mechanical properties and controlled degradation kinetics. By blending these constituents, biocomposites achieve synergistic properties: the biological cues of natural ECM mimetics coupled with the mechanical robustness of synthetic scaffolds. Collagen–hydroxyapatite (HAp) composites exemplify bone-mimetic biocomposites. Collagen provides a fibrous network fostering osteoblast adhesion and proliferation, whereas HAp delivers osteoconductivity and mechanical stiffness approximating trabecular bone (~ 50–150 MPa compressive modulus). Similarly, PCL–collagen composites have been tailored for cartilage engineering, achieving compressive moduli (~ 10 MPa) similar to native articular cartilage (6–20 MPa) and supporting chondrocyte differentiation. Chitosan–alginate hydrogels, which form polyelectrolyte networks, have been widely employed as lungs, skin, and vascular tissue substitutes due to their high water content (> 90%), tunable viscoelasticity ($G' \approx 0.5$–1 kPa), and amenability to cell encapsulation [62].

Biocomposite fabrication techniques are equally diverse. Solvent casting/porogen leaching (SCPL) permits precise pore size control (100–300 μm) for bone and cartilage scaffolds, yet residual solvents may hamper cell viability if not thoroughly removed. Electrospinning yields nanofibrous mats (fiber diameters 50–500 nm) that mimic collagen fibrils, directing fibroblast and endothelial cell alignment for skin and vascular engineering, respectively. Three-dimensional (3D) printing enables patient-specific, biomimetic geometries with graded porosities and multi-material deposition; for instance, extrusion-based printing of PLA–HAp composites has produced scaffolds with ~ 70% porosity and interconnectivity, facilitating vascular ingrowth in vivo. In situ polymerization (e.g., photoinitiated crosslinking of gelatin methacryloyl [GelMA]) allows minimally invasive scaffold formation in irregular defect cavities, promoting direct integration with surrounding tissue. Functionalization strategies further refine biocomposite performance. Grafting RGD peptides onto PCL–HAp scaffolds enhances mesenchymal stem cell (MSC) adhesion by ~ 2.5-fold without significant loss in mechanical stiffness (~ 55 MPa), while heparin-based coatings sequester growth factors (e.g., FGF-2, VEGF) to promote angiogenesis and osteogenesis in a spatiotemporally controlled manner. Smart biocomposites, incorporating thermoresponsive poly(N-isopropylacrylamide) (PNIPAAm) or enzyme-sensitive linkers (e.g., MMP-cleavable peptides), adapt their degradation or drug-release profiles to local physiological cues, enhancing on-demand tissue regeneration.

Preclinical evaluations demonstrate promising results across various tissue types. In rat cranial defect models, collagen–HAp scaffolds seeded with MSCs achieved ~ 85% defect closure and robust new bone volume (BV/TV ~ 45%) at 12 weeks, compared to ~ 35% in acellular controls. Chitosan–alginate hydrogels loaded with keratinocytes accelerated wound closure in diabetic murine models, reducing healing time by ~ 30% relative to standard dressings. PCL–collagen–elastin vascular grafts exhibited 80% patency and uniform endothelialization in a canine carotid model at 6 months, indicating potential for small-diameter vascular reconstructions. Despite significant progress, challenges remain: matching mechanical properties without sacrificing bioactivity, controlling degradation rates to align with native tissue healing (e.g., bone: 6–12 months; cartilage: 8–12 weeks; skin: 4–6 weeks), and ensuring long-term immunocompatibility [16]. However, leveraging advanced fabrication (e.g., multi-material 3D bioprinting), functionalization (e.g., dual-growth factor delivery), and computational modeling (finite element analysis for mechanical prediction) continues to mitigate these obstacles.

In summary, biocomposites in artificial tissue engineering bridge the gap between purely synthetic scaffolds and natural ECM analogs, delivering tailored mechanical support and biological functionality. Their modular design, combined with evolving processing techniques, positions them at the forefront of next-generation regenerative therapies [63].

6.8.2 *Future Potential in Regenerative Medicine*

Biocomposites hold enormous promise for advancing regenerative medicine by providing customizable, biologically active scaffolds that actively participate in tissue repair. Personalized medicine is a near-term application: patient-specific biocomposites, manufactured via 3D bioprinting from autologous cells and biomaterials, can minimize immune rejection and enhance integration. For example, coupling patient-derived induced pluripotent stem cells (iPSCs) with a biodegradable PLA–collagen ink allowed printing of cartilage constructs that exhibited ~ 85% viability and chondrogenic marker expression (SOX9) after 21 days in vitro. In vivo, these constructs achieved 70% restoration of mechanical properties (compressive modulus ~ 8 MPa) in a large-animal (sheep) knee defect model at 12 weeks.

Organ-on-Chip (OoC) Integration with biocomposites offers another horizon. Biocomposite hydrogels (e.g., PEG–gelatin–HAp) incorporating microfluidic vascular channels can recapitulate physiological flow and dynamic mechanical cues, enhancing tissue maturation. A liver-mimetic OoC with a GelMA–HAp scaffold achieved albumin secretion levels comparable to native liver (~2.5 μg/h/million cells) over 14 days, outperforming 2D cultures by ~ threefold. Such platforms can accelerate drug screening, reduce reliance on animal models, and personalize therapies (e.g., patient-specific drug toxicity profiling).

Smart, Responsive Biocomposites that adapt to local cues can further revolutionize treatment paradigms. Enzyme-responsive hydrogels engineered to release anti-fibrotic agents upon detecting elevated matrix metalloproteinase-9 (MMP-9) levels in myocardial infarction sites reduced fibrotic scar size by ~ 35% in rat models, improving ejection fraction by ~ 15% at 8 weeks compared to untreated controls [41]. Similarly, pH-sensitive composites loaded with anti-inflammatory drugs deliver therapeutics only under acidic inflammatory conditions ($pH < 6.8$), minimizing systemic side effects. In a diabetic wound model, such a scaffold accelerated wound closure by ~ 50% and decreased pro-inflammatory cytokines (IL-6) by ~ 40% relative to nonresponsive hydrogels [64].

Integration with Gene and Cell Therapies presents additional avenues. Biocomposite scaffolds can serve as localized gene delivery platforms. Polyurethane–gelatin scaffolds functionalized with lentiviral vectors encoding VEGF achieved sustained VEGF expression in vivo, increasing capillary density by ~ 60% in ischemic limb models [43]. Incorporating CRISPR/Cas9 plasmids into a chitosan–PLGA composite allowed site-specific gene editing in resident fibroblasts, downregulating pro-fibrotic TGF-β1 expression by ~ 70% and reducing scar tissue formation by ~ 45% in rat skin wounds.

Bioprinting Vascularized Tissues remains a critical frontier. Perfusable vascular networks within biocomposite constructs are essential for nutrient delivery beyond 200 μm depths. Using digital light processing (DLP) 3D printing of GelMA–HAp composite inks, researchers fabricated microchannels (100 μm diameter) lined with endothelial cells that achieved 80% patency and stable lumens under 10 dyn/cm^2 shear stress in vitro [45]. Transplantation into immunodeficient mice formed functional microvasculature within 2 weeks, with 75% microvessel perfusion as measured by lectin perfusion assays.

Neural Tissue Engineering also stands to benefit. Biocomposite conduits combining PCL–collagen and aligned electrospun fibers loaded with nerve growth factor (NGF) facilitated peripheral nerve regeneration across 15 mm sciatic nerve gaps in rats, achieving compound muscle action potentials (CMAP) at ~ 75% of contralateral healthy nerves by 16 weeks [47]. Incorporating conductive polymers (polypyrrole) into these conduits allowed electrical stimulation (50 mV/mm), doubling axonal outgrowth rates (~ 1.2 mm/day vs. ~ 0.6 mm/day without stimulation).

Clinical Translation will hinge on addressing scalability, cost, and regulatory challenges. Economies of scale and modular manufacturing platforms (e.g., multi-nozzle bioprinters in GMP facilities) can reduce unit costs by ~ 40%. Allogeneic "off-the-shelf" biocomposite patches for diabetic foot ulcers have entered Phase II trials, demonstrating safety and a 30% increase in healing rates compared to standard care. Combined with streamlined regulatory pathways (e.g., EMA's adaptive access), biocomposites are poised for rapid clinical adoption.

Ultimately, biocomposites converge material science, tissue biology, and engineering to enable next-generation regenerative therapies—ranging from patient-specific grafts and organoids to responsive drug-delivery implants—ushering in a new era of personalized, effective, and cost-efficient treatments.

References

1. Valente KP, Brolo A, Suleman A (2020) From dermal patch to implants—applications of biocomposites in living tissues. Molecules 25:507
2. Gupta S, Gupta V, Chanda A (2022) Biomechanical modeling of novel high expansion auxetic skin grafts. Int J Numer Method Biomed Eng 38:e3586
3. Ellahi A, Gupta S, Bose D, Chanda A (2025) A high-fidelity biomechanical modeling framework for injury prediction during frontal car crash. Comput Methods Biomech Biomed Eng 28:13–24
4. Viola M et al (2021) The importance of interfaces in multi-material biofabricated tissue structures. Adv Healthc Mater 10:2101021
5. Modrák M, Trebuňová M, Balogová AF, Hudák R, Živčák J (2023) Biodegradable materials for tissue engineering: development, classification and current applications. J Funct Biomater 14:159
6. Liu S et al (2023) Biomimetic natural biomaterials for tissue engineering and regenerative medicine: new biosynthesis methods, recent advances, and emerging applications. Mil Med Res 10(1):1–30
7. Vivcharenko V et al (2025) Application of hydroxyapatite composites in bone tissue engineering: a review. J Funct Biomater 16:127
8. Wahl DA, Czernuszka JT (2006) Collagen-hydroxyapatite composites for hard tissue repair. Eur Cells Mater 11:43–56
9. Chanda A, Gupta S (2025) Healthcare entrepreneurship and management. Routledge, Taylor & Francis Group
10. Singla R, Gupta S, Chanda A (2023) A computational fluid dynamics-based model for assessing rupture risk in cerebral arteries with varying aneurysm sizes. Math Comput Appl 28:90
11. Low SP, Williams KA, Canham LT, Voelcker NH (2006) Evaluation of mammalian cell adhesion on surface-modified porous silicon. Biomaterials 27:4538–4546
12. Petricca SE, Marra KG, Kumta PN (2006) Chemical synthesis of poly(lactic-co-glycolic acid)/hydroxyapatite composites for orthopaedic applications. Acta Biomater 2:277–286
13. Abdallah MN et al (2017) Biomaterial surface proteomic signature determines interaction with epithelial cells. Acta Biomater 54:150–163
14. Martino MM et al (2011) Engineering the growth factor microenvironment with fibronectin domains to promote wound and bone tissue healing. Sci Transl Med 3
15. Gupta S, Singh G, Chanda A (2021) Prediction of diabetic foot ulcer progression: a computational study. Biomed Phys Eng Express 7:065020
16. Wei S, Ma JX, Xu L, Gu XS, Ma XL (2020) Biodegradable materials for bone defect repair. Mil Med Res 7(1):1–25
17. Garcia-Garcia A et al (2024) Biodegradable natural hydrogels for tissue engineering, controlled release, and soil remediation. Polymers 16:2599
18. Yadav P, Kamboj M, Das B (2024) Application of nanotechnology in antimicrobial coating on surgical instruments. Appl Nanotechnol Biomed Eng 150–168. https://doi.org/10.1201/978 1003432661-9

19. Majhy B, Priyadarshini P, Sen AK (2021) Effect of surface energy and roughness on cell adhesion and growth—facile surface modification for enhanced cell culture. RSC Adv 11:15467
20. Singh G, Yadav P, Chanda A (2024) Development of biofidelic skin simulants based on fresh cadaveric skin tests. Eur Burn J 5:454–463
21. Yadav P et al (2025) Gelatin multiwalled carbon nanotube composite 3D printed semi biological mesh for abdominal hernia treatment. Chem Asian J 20:e202401136
22. Verma S, Chanda A (2024) State-of-the-art of finite element modelling of the human spine to study the impact of vibrations: a review. Int J Comput Methods Eng Sci Mech 25:225–247
23. Verma S, Singh G, Chanda A (2023) A novel finite element model for the study of harmful vibrations on the aging spine. Computation 11:93
24. Verma S, Singh G, Chanda A (2024) Development of a computational framework for determination of detrimental vibrations on the human spine segments. Multiscale Sci Eng 61(6):48–56
25. Chanda A, Chatterjee S, Gupta V (2020) Soft composite based hyperelastic model for anisotropic tissue characterization. J Compos Mater 54:4525–4534
26. Chanda A, Unnikrishnan V, Flynn Z, Lackey K (2017) Experimental study on tissue phantoms to understand the effect of injury and suturing on human skin mechanical properties. Proc Inst Mech Eng Part H J Eng Med 231:80–91
27. Seid AM, Adimass SA (2024) Review on the impact behavior of natural fiber epoxy based composites. Heliyon 10:e39116
28. Gentleman E et al (2003) Mechanical characterization of collagen fibers and scaffolds for tissue engineering. Biomaterials 24:3805–3813
29. Chanda A, Upchurch W (2018) Biomechanical modeling of wounded skin. J Compos Sci 2:69
30. Singh G, Chanda A (2024) Development and biomechanical testing of artificial surrogates for vaginal tissue. Adv Mater Process Technol. https://doi.org/10.1080/2374068X.2023.2198837
31. Gupta V, Singh G, Chanda A (2024) Modeling of metamaterial based incision patterns for generating high expansions in skin grafts. Lect Notes Mech Eng 563–574. https://doi.org/10.1007/978-981-99-5919-8_51
32. Fitzgerald A et al (2021) A life cycle engineering perspective on biocomposites as a solution for a sustainable recovery. Sustainability 13:1160
33. Solechan S et al (2023) Characterization of PLA/PCL/nano-hydroxyapatite (nHA) biocomposites prepared via cold isostatic pressing. Polymers 15:559
34. Shanbhag S et al (2021) Bone regeneration in rat calvarial defects using dissociated or spheroid mesenchymal stromal cells in scaffold-hydrogel constructs. Stem Cell Res Ther 12:575
35. Singh G, Chanda A (2022) Biomechanical modeling of progressive wound healing: a computational study. Biomed Eng Adv 4:100055
36. Bose D, Gupta S, Chanda A (2025) Scalable direct manufacturing of a functional multipurpose wrist-hand orthosis using 3D printing. Ann 3D Print Med 17:100186
37. Chhikara K, Gupta S, Chanda A (2022) Development of a novel foot orthosis for plantar pain reduction. Mater Today Proc 62:3532–3537
38. Naik A, Shepherd DV, Shepherd JH, Best SM, Cameron RE (2017) The effect of the type of HA on the degradation of PLGA/HA composites. Mater Sci Eng C 70:824–831
39. Dias JR, Sousa A, Augusto A, Bártolo PJ, Granja PL (2022) Electrospun polycaprolactone (PCL) degradation: an in vitro and in vivo study. Polymers 14:3397
40. Chen Z et al (2024) Degradation behaviors of polylactic acid, polyglycolic acid, and their copolymer films in simulated marine environments. Polymers (Basel) 16:1765
41. Chhikara K, Gupta S, Bose D, Kataria C, Chanda A (2023) Development and trial of a multipurpose customized orthosis for activities of daily living in patients with spinal cord injury. Prosthesis 5:467–479
42. Rothschild BM et al (2023) Design, manufacturing, and trial of a 3D printed customized finger splint for patients with rheumatoid arthritis. Rheumato 3:51–62
43. Chhikara K, Sidhu SS, Gupta S, Saharawat S, Kataria C, Chanda A (2023) Development and effectiveness testing of a novel 3D-printed multi-material orthosis in nurses with plantar foot pain. Prosthesis 5:73–87

44. ISO 10993-1:2018 Biological evaluation of medical devices—Part 1: evaluation and testing within a risk management process. https://www.iso.org/standard/68936.html
45. Hennessy KM et al (2008) The effect of RGD peptides on osseointegration of hydroxyapatite biomaterials. Biomaterials 29:3075–3083
46. Deepthi S, Jeevitha K, Nivedhitha Sundaram M, Chennazhi KP, Jayakumar R (2015) Chitosan–hyaluronic acid hydrogel coated poly(caprolactone) multiscale bilayer scaffold for ligament regeneration. Chem Eng J 260:478–485
47. Kumar VB, Tiwari OS, Finkelstein-Zuta G, Rencus-Lazar S, Gazit E (2023) Design of functional RGD peptide-based biomaterials for tissue engineering. Pharmaceutics 15:345
48. Anti-CD44 antibody—mesenchymal stem cell marker (ab157107) | Abcam. https://www.abcam.com/en-us/products/primary-antibodies/cd44-antibody-ab157107?srsltid=AfmBOorYXbS-y12WAzaSSMg5mNHKJmW_yzPG247kgO6KcUI1PLnCWRuo
49. Dai M et al (2024) Antibacterial sequential growth factor delivery from alginate/gelatin methacryloyl microspheres for bone regeneration. Int J Biol Macromol 275:133557
50. Ansari MJ et al (2022) Poly(N-isopropylacrylamide)-based hydrogels for biomedical applications: a review of the state-of-the-art. Gels 8:454
51. Singh G, Gupta V, Chanda A (2022) Mechanical characterization of rotating triangle shaped auxetic skin graft simulants. Facta Univ Ser Mech Eng
52. Gupta V, Singh G, Chanda A, Chanda A (2021) Expansion potential of skin grafts with novel I-shaped auxetic incisions. Biomed Phys Eng Express 8:015016
53. Singh G, Gupta V, Chanda A (2022) Artificial skin with varying biomechanical properties. Mater Today Proc 62:3162–3166
54. Jiang C et al (2022) Biomechanics of skin grafts: effect of pattern size, spacing and orientation. Eng Res Express 4:015006
55. Singh G, Chanda A (2024) Finite element modeling of diabetic foot: a state-of-the-art review. Eng Res Express 6:012507
56. Gupta V, Singh G, Chanda A (2023) Development of hierarchical auxetic skin graft simulants with high expansion potential. Biomed Eng Adv 5:100087
57. Maia FR, Lourenço AH, Granja PL, Gonçalves RM, Barrias CC (2014) Effect of cell density on mesenchymal stem cells aggregation in RGD-alginate 3D matrices under osteoinductive conditions. Macromol Biosci 14:759–771
58. Gupta V, Singla R, Chanda A (2023) Development and characterization of novel anisotropic skin graft simulants. Dermato 3:114–130
59. Gupta V, Chanda A (2023) Auxetic incisions with alternating slit shapes: a promising technique for enhancing synthetic skin grafts expansion. Mater Res Express 10:075802
60. Gupta V, Gupta S, Chanda A (2023) Development of an ultra-low-cost planar biaxial tester for soft tissue characterization. Biomed Phys Eng Express 9:025011
61. Ornelas-González A, González-González M, Rito-Palomares M (2021) Microcarrier-based stem cell bioprocessing: GMP-grade culture challenges and future trends for regenerative medicine. Crit Rev Biotechnol 41:1081–1095
62. Malda J et al (2013) 25th anniversary article: engineering hydrogels for biofabrication. Adv Mater 25:5011–5028
63. Turnbull G et al (2018) 3D bioactive composite scaffolds for bone tissue engineering. Bioact Mater 3:278–314
64. Zarur M, Seijo-Rabina A, Goyanes A, Concheiro A, Alvarez-Lorenzo C (2023) PH-responsive scaffolds for tissue regeneration: in vivo performance. Acta Biomater 168:22–41

Chapter 7
Hydrogels-Based Artificial Tissues

Each year, millions of patients experience organ or tissue loss due to illness or injury, requiring over 8 million surgeries annually in the U.S., with costs exceeding $400 billion. While organ and tissue transplantation is an effective treatment, a severe donor shortage limits its availability [1]. For instance, although heart transplants could benefit nearly 40,000 patients annually, only 2300 were performed in 1997, according to the American Heart Association. Similarly, over 10,000 patients need skin grafts each year for severe burns or skin cancer in the US, further emphasizing the gap between demand and available resources [2]. The development of artificial organs and tissues presents an innovative approach to addressing the need for transplants. A notable method combines a patient's own cells with polymer scaffolds to engineer new tissues. The process begins by isolating tissue-specific cells from a small patient sample, which are then cultured and integrated into 3D polymer scaffolds. These scaffolds mimic the natural extracellular matrix, supporting cell growth and guiding the formation of new tissue. They also help deliver cells to the target site and can influence the shape and function of the engineered tissue [3, 4]. This technique has been applied to create various tissues, including artificial arteries, bladders, skin, cartilage, bones, ligaments, and tendons. Many of these engineered tissues are already being used or are close to clinical application, demonstrating their therapeutic potential [5–7].

Furthermore, strategies are being explored to induce specific cell types and functions, either by differentiating mature cells or directing the behavior of stem cells. This approach holds promise for regenerative medicine, offering personalized treatments that minimize rejection risks and improve patient outcomes. Polymer scaffolds are essential in tissue engineering, as they replicate the functions of natural extracellular matrices (ECMs). ECMs, made of amino acids and sugar-based polymers, provide structural support, regulate cellular activity, and facilitate the transport of nutrients, metabolites, and growth factors [8]. Various polymers have been explored for use in tissue engineering [9], with synthetic aliphatic polyesters such as poly(glycolic acid) (PGA), poly(lactic acid) (PLA), and their copolymers (PLGA) being the most widely

A. Chanda and D. Sharma, *Handbook of Artificial Tissues, Biofabrication and Bioprinting, Volume I*, Biomedical Materials for Multi-functional Applications,
https://doi.org/10.1007/978-981-92-1307-8_7

used. These materials are FDA-approved and have a proven track record in medical applications. However, their implantation requires surgeons to make large incisions to fit the polymer scaffolds, which can pose challenges during surgical procedures. Injectable polymers, especially hydrogels, present an innovative and less invasive option for delivering cells in tissue engineering. These materials are biocompatible and structurally similar to the body's natural macromolecules, making them ideal for medical use. Hydrogels have a long history in drug delivery and are now being utilized as scaffolds to support the development of new tissues in tissue engineering [10].

This chapter discusses the key design parameters of hydrogels for tissue engineering applications. Hydrogels, whether in current use or under consideration, are categorized into two groups based on their composition: synthetic and natural. Natural polymer hydrogels have been widely used in tissue engineering, but their limitations have led to efforts to modify them and incorporate various synthetic polymers. Synthetic polymers offer favorable chemical and physical properties for these applications. The paper also explores future directions, including the use of mechanical stimuli to enhance tissue growth and the incorporation of growth factors [11].

7.1 Design Specification of Hydrogel in Tissue Engineering

For hydrogels to be effective in tissue engineering and support the growth of new tissue, they must meet several important design criteria. These include biological factors, such as cell adhesion, and physical properties, such as degradation and mechanical strength. A critical factor is biocompatibility, which means the material must be able to function in the body without causing harm to nearby cells, excessive scarring, or negative reactions that hinder its intended purpose. This is especially important because the immune response to the transplanted cells can be influenced by the inflammatory reaction to the hydrogel. While synthetic polymers may cause adverse reactions in the body, natural polymers typically offer better biocompatibility [12, 13]. This creates some limitations when using synthetic polymers to design hydrogels for various applications. Another important factor to consider is the gelling process, which can involve ionic or covalent crosslinking, as well as intrinsic phase transition behavior. Hydrogels can be easily formed through ion crosslinking using multivalent counterions, but in aqueous environments, these ions can exchange with other ionic molecules, leading to uncontrolled degradation of the hydrogel's original properties. A common method to regulate the crosslinking density of hydrogels is covalent crosslinking [14].

However, creating non-degradable crosslinks can be problematic for most tissue engineering applications, and the toxicity of crosslinking agents must also be considered. The mechanical properties of hydrogels are critical design factors in tissue engineering, as they must create and maintain a suitable space for tissue formation. These properties are also closely tied to cell adhesion and gene expression. The primary factors influencing the mechanical characteristics of hydrogels include the stiffness of polymer chains, the type and density of crosslinking molecules, and the swelling behavior resulting from the balance between hydrophilicity and hydrophobicity [15]. In tissue engineering, controlled degradation of the hydrogel is also essential, whether it is made from synthetic or natural materials. The degradation rate should align with the pace of tissue growth, which varies depending on the type of tissue being produced. Hydrogels can degrade through processes like hydrolysis, enzyme activity, or dissolution. Typically, the mechanical properties and degradation rate of crosslinked gels are related. However, by intentionally introducing flaws into the network, these properties can sometimes be decoupled, leading to softer hydrogels that degrade more slowly than stiffer, more highly crosslinked gels. One approach to forming hydrogels is utilizing the phase transition properties of certain polymers. For example, a polymer solution can transition into a gel with a slight temperature change around the lower critical solution temperature (LCST). Much research has focused on controlling the LCST to make it align with body temperature. Additionally, in orthopedic tissue engineering, hydrogels have been developed that are crosslinked in situ with minimal temperature increase during polymerization. Cell adhesion, migration, and differentiation are significantly influenced by their interactions with hydrogels. The adhesion process, which may vary by cell type, is often determined by the interaction between specific cell receptors and ligands present in or adsorbed onto the materials. Inappropriate interactions could lead to undesirable tissue formation [16].

7.2 Materials for Gel Formation

Hydrogels used as scaffolds in tissue engineering can be derived from various synthetic and natural materials. Synthetic options include poly(ethylene oxide) (PEO), poly(vinyl alcohol) (PVA), poly(acrylic acid) (PAA), poly(propylene fumarate-co-ethylene glycol) (P(PF-co-EG)), and polypeptides. Natural polymers include agarose, alginate, chitosan, collagen, fibrin, gelatin, and hyaluronic acid (HA). Due to their prevalent use in tissue engineering, this section focuses on a selected group of these hydrogels: PEO, PVA, P(PF-co-EG), alginate, chitosan, collagen, and HA. It covers their chemical properties, gelling conditions, and degradation mechanisms.

7.2.1 Synthetic Materials

Synthetic hydrogels are highly valued in tissue engineering due to their consistent and controllable properties. Synthetic polymers can be engineered with specific molecular weights, block structures, degradable bonds, and crosslinking mechanisms, influencing their crosslinking density, gel formation, mechanical strength, and degradation behavior. Examples of synthetic hydrogels include poly(ethylene oxide) (PEO), poly(vinyl alcohol) (PVA), and poly(propylene fumarate-co-ethylene glycol) (P(PF-co-EG)). PEO, widely used in tissue engineering and FDA-approved for various medical applications, is a hydrophilic polymer chemically similar to polyethylene glycol (PEG). By modifying PEO or PEG with acrylates or methacrylates and using UV light with a photoinitiator, hydrogels can be formed. Block copolymers of PEO or PEG with poly(l-lactic acid) (PLLA) are used to produce thermally reversible hydrogels. Additionally, degradable hydrogels can be synthesized using hydrolytically degradable poly(lactic acid) (PLA) or enzyme-cleavable oligopeptides. PVA is another synthetic polymer extensively studied for drug delivery and space-filling applications [17].

The semi-transparent PVA/PEG gel is applied to a nonwoven fabric, as shown in Fig. 7.1a. The mechanical properties of the PVA/PEG gel enhanced with GO nanoparticles significantly surpass those of the PVA/PEG hydrogel, exhibiting a breaking strain of $120 \pm 10\%$ and a breaking strength of 20 ± 5 kPa. The black cylindrical sample depicted in Fig. 7.1b demonstrates the transformation of the composite hydrogel into a stable, highly elastic black form upon incorporating GO nanoparticles into PVA/PEGsol. At 1000× magnification, Fig. 7.1c vividly captures the morphology of the black hydrogel after it has been cooled and dried, leaving only the polymeric skeleton. The porous nature of the hydrogel skeleton is evident, with water molecules occupying the pores when hydrated. As illustrated in Fig. 7.1d, the cavity walls are exceptionally thin, and the internal voids are interconnected by narrow, "nozzle-shaped" throats. Additionally, smaller porous sheet-like networks within each pore form porous walls, enhancing resistance to ion transport [18]. Hydrogels from PVA can be formed through chemical crosslinking with agents like glutaraldehyde or physically by repeated freeze–thaw cycles. These versatile properties make synthetic hydrogels an appealing choice for various tissue engineering applications. Hyaluronic acid (HA) hydrogels are formed through covalent crosslinking methods such as hydrazide derivatives, esterification, and annealing [19].

Composite hydrogels have also been developed by combining HA with other polymers like alginate and collagen. Since HA is naturally degraded by hyaluronidase, its breakdown can be regulated by cells in the body, enabling localized control over material degradation. Alginate is widely used in medical applications, including cell encapsulation and drug delivery, due to its mild gelling conditions, low toxicity, and abundant availability [20]. Derived from bacteria and brown seaweed, alginate is a linear polysaccharide made of (1–4)-linked β-d-mannuronic acid (M) and α-l-guluronic acid (G) monomers. These monomers are arranged in repetitive or alternating blocks within the polymer. The specific composition of alginate varies

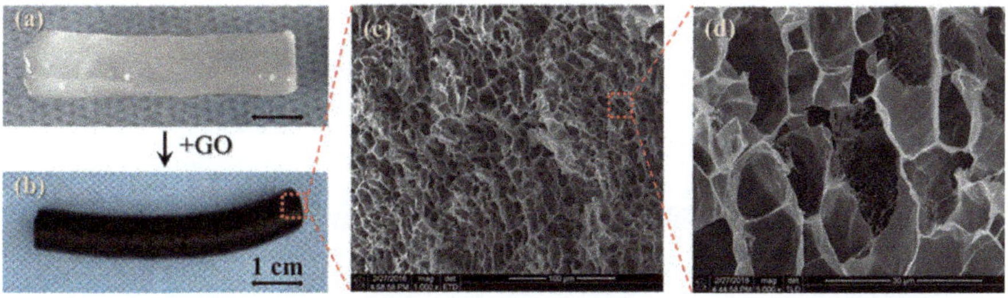

Fig. 7.1 Hydrogel samples: **a** PVA/PEG and **b** PVA/PEG/GO. SEM images reveal the porous structure of the gel in its cooled and dried states, with **c** shown at 1000× magnification and **d** depicting a small section of (**c**) at 5000× magnification. Figure reproduced under license CC-BY-4.0 [18] (https://creativecommons.org/licenses/by/4.0/)

based on the species, location, and age of the seaweed source. Gels form when divalent cations, such as Ca^{2+}, Ba^{2+}, or Sr^{2+}, create ionic bridges between G monomer blocks across polymer chains. By adjusting the M-to-G ratio, the crosslinking density, mechanical properties, and pore size of the gels can be controlled, making alginate hydrogels highly versatile for tissue engineering and biomedical use [21]. PVA can also be combined with other water-soluble polymers and crosslinked through chemical or physical methods, resulting in forms that are insoluble in aqueous solutions. A newer synthetic block copolymer, poly(propylene fumarate-co-ethylene glycol) (P(PF-co-EG)), has been developed as an injectable carrier for applications in vascular and bone tissue engineering. Poly(propylene fumarate) (PPF), a hydrophobic, linear polyester, degrades through hydrolysis of its ester bonds. When PPF is copolymerized with hydrophilic PEG and crosslinked either chemically or via UV light exposure, it forms hydrogels suitable for biomedical use [22, 23].

7.2.2 Naturally Derived Materials

Naturally derived hydrogels are widely used in tissue engineering due to their compatibility with the natural extracellular matrix (ECM). Collagen, the primary structural protein in the ECM, makes up about 25% of total protein in mammals and is abundant in mammalian tissues [24]. Hyaluronic acid (HA) is also present in varying concentrations across all mature animal tissues. Natural carbohydrate polymers (NCPs) are long-chain polymers composed of sugar monomers connected by glycosidic bonds. These polymers are widely available in nature, renewable, non-toxic, and generally non-immunogenic. They exhibit strong water affinity, biocompatibility, and biodegradability, making them excellent base materials for hydrogels in biomedical applications. Furthermore, their chemical structure allows for extensive modifications, enabling customization of their properties to suit specific purposes shown in Fig. 7.2 [25].

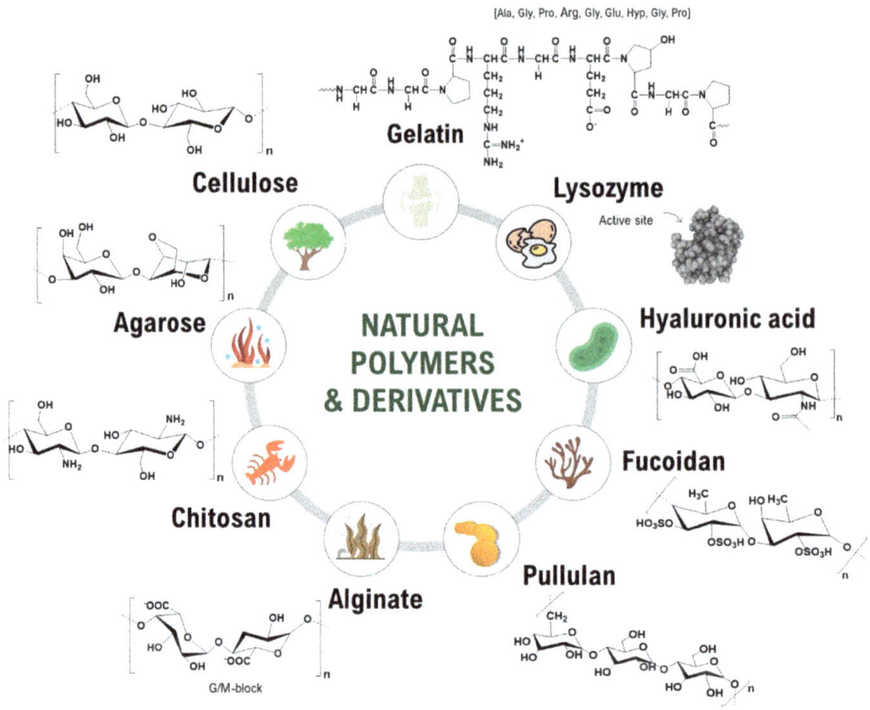

Fig. 7.2 Natural hydrogels are derived from carbohydrate polymers found in nature. Figure reproduced under license CC-BY-4.0 [25] (https://creativecommons.org/licenses/by/4.0/)

Similar to HA, alginate and chitosan are hydrophilic, linear polysaccharides that have shown favorable in vivo interactions, making them effective hydrogel scaffold materials [21, 26]. Collagen's widespread presence and role as a key ECM component make it highly attractive for biomedical applications. It consists of three polypeptide chains forming a triple-helix structure, held together by covalent and hydrogen bonds. These collagen strands can self-aggregate into stable fibers. Collagen scaffolds can be further strengthened through chemical crosslinking using agents like glutaraldehyde, formaldehyde, or carbodiimide, as well as through physical methods such as UV irradiation, freeze-drying, and heating. Blending collagen with other polymers, such as HA, PLA, PGA, PLGA, chitosan, and PEO [27, 28] also enhances its mechanical properties. Collagen is naturally degraded by metalloproteases, including collagenase and serine proteases, allowing for controlled breakdown by cells in engineered tissues. This localized degradation helps regulate scaffold remodeling, supporting tissue growth and integration. Overall, collagen's versatility and biocompatibility make it a valuable material for developing hydrogels and scaffolds in tissue engineering. Hyaluronic acid (HA), the simplest glycosaminoglycan (GAG), is present in nearly all mammalian tissues and fluids, particularly abundant in joint synovial fluid and during wound healing [29]. It is a linear polymer composed of repeating disaccharides and varies in molecular weight. Alginate, another natural polymer, can form hydrogels through ionic or covalent crosslinking. Covalent crosslinking involves carbodiimide chemistry with agents like adipic hydrazide and PEG. Ionically crosslinked alginate hydrogels gradually dissolve rather than degrade, losing mechanical stiffness due to calcium ion exchange and chain dissociation [30].

Modified forms such as oxidized alginate and poly(aldehyde guluronate) (PAG) enable hydrolytic degradation. Chitosan, structurally similar to natural GAGs, is derived from chitin found in arthropod exoskeletons. It consists of (1–4)-linked d-glucosamine and N-acetyl-d-glucosamine units. The degree of N-deacetylation, typically between 50 and 90%, influences its crystallinity, with maximum crystallinity at 0% or 100% deacetylation. Chitosan dissolves in dilute acids that protonate its free amino groups. It can be gelled by extrusion into a nonsolvent or by increasing the pH. Crosslinking methods such as glutaraldehyde treatment, UV irradiation, and temperature changes are also used to form chitosan gels and derivatives. Chitosan is broken down by lysozyme, with the degradation rate inversely related to its crystallinity. These properties make HA, alginate, and chitosan valuable materials for various tissue engineering applications [31–34].

7.3 Variables in Scaffold Design

The selection or synthesis of hydrogel scaffold materials depends on the physical properties, mass transport capabilities, and biological interactions required for a specific application. These design considerations are influenced by the intended use of the scaffold and the environment in which it will be implanted. For example, scaffolds designed for cell encapsulation must facilitate the diffusion of nutrients and metabolites between the encapsulated cells and surrounding tissue, form gels without damaging the cells, remain non-toxic post-gelling, and possess sufficient mechanical strength to withstand implantation and in vivo conditions. In this context, diffusion needs to dictate mass transport properties, while mechanical strength and gel formation dynamics depend on physical characteristics. Additionally, the requirement for non-toxicity highlights the importance of biological properties. This discussion focuses on the key physical, mass transport, and biological design parameters essential for developing hydrogel scaffolds in tissue engineering [35–38].

7.3.1 Physical Properties

Scaffolds in tissue engineering provide a framework for tissue regeneration by initially occupying spaces meant for natural tissue. The physical characteristics of these scaffolds, such as mechanical properties, degradation behavior, and gel formation dynamics, are crucial to their performance. These attributes are influenced by the main polymer structure, crosslinking properties, and environmental conditions.

Hydrogels, commonly used as scaffolds, offer unique advantages due to their ability to form gels in situ. The kinetics of gel formation play a critical role in incorporating cells and bioactive molecules into the scaffold and controlling their delivery. However, traditional scaffold formation methods involving changes in temperature, pH, or solvents may damage proteins and cells. To avoid this, scaffolds can be preformed before adding bioactive agents. Interestingly, some hydrogels can be mixed with cells and bioactive compounds prior to injection, forming gels in vivo without harming the embedded materials. Examples of such hydrogels include polyethylene oxide (PEO), chitosan, in vivo gelling alginate, and P(PF-co-EG). Success in this approach relies on controlling gelation speed and flow properties, ensuring the scaffold is formed efficiently and safely in the body [39–42]. The mechanical properties of scaffolds at both macro and micro levels are critical for effective tissue engineering. At the macroscopic level, scaffolds must withstand stress to maintain volume and provide stability during tissue formation. On the microscopic scale, mechanical stimuli are essential for cell proliferation, differentiation, and overall tissue development. Therefore, scaffolds must be able to bear loads and appropriately transfer mechanical forces to cells and surrounding tissues [43, 44]. Key mechanical properties, including elasticity, compressibility, viscoelasticity, tensile strength, and failure strain, must be carefully specified, characterized, and controlled to ensure optimal scaffold performance. These properties in hydrogels are influenced by factors such as polymer composition, crosslinking density, swelling, and environmental conditions like pH and temperature. For instance, the mechanical strength and compression modulus of alginate hydrogels increase with a higher ratio of G to M subunits and longer G-blocks [21]. Increasing the alginate concentration from 1 to 3% also enhances its compression modulus and shear modulus. Similar trends are observed in PVA and PEG hydrogels, where a higher weight fraction of PEG (from 10 to 40%) improves mechanical strength [44, 45].

Crosslinking plays a significant role in determining a hydrogel's mechanical properties. Ionically crosslinked alginate hydrogels gain strength with higher ion concentration and the use of divalent ions with greater affinity for alginate. In covalently crosslinked hydrogels, adjusting crosslinker type and density can independently regulate mechanical properties and swelling behavior [46]. Generally, swelling reduces hydrogel strength, and degradation further weakens the material unless compensated by tissue ingrowth or specific modifications that decouple these effects. The ideal degradation kinetics of scaffolds in tissue engineering depend on the specific application. In scenarios involving the controlled release of molecules or functional tissue regeneration, degradation is essential. However, in applications like cell encapsulation for immunoisolation, degradation may not be necessary. The scaffold's degradation rate should ideally match tissue formation rates or allow for the controlled release of bioactive compounds [47–49]. Understanding and controlling degradation processes are crucial. Hydrogels typically degrade through hydrolysis, enzymatic cleavage, or dissolution. Synthetic materials, such as PEG-PLA copolymers, degrade via hydrolysis of ester bonds at a consistent rate regardless of environmental conditions. Enzymatic degradation, which affects materials like collagen, hyaluronic acid (HA), and chitosan, depends on the availability of enzymes and the number of cleavage sites in the polymer. Modifications, such as synthetic linkages in polyethylene oxide (PEO), can render it susceptible to enzymatic breakdown. Ionically crosslinked alginate usually dissolves in response to its ionic environment but can also undergo controlled hydrolysis after oxidation. The dissolution rate of alginate depends on the local ionic conditions. By tailoring these degradation mechanisms, scaffold breakdown can be synchronized with tissue formation or molecule release, optimizing the scaffold's performance for various applications.

7.3.2 Mass Transport Properties

The effectiveness of scaffolds in tissue engineering relies heavily on the proper transport of gases, nutrients, proteins, cells, and waste. Initially, diffusion is the primary mechanism of mass transport. The rate and distance of molecular diffusion within a scaffold are influenced by the material's properties and the interactions between molecules and the scaffold's nanoporous structure. Key factors affecting this structure include crosslinker concentration, polymer size, and polymer fraction. Diffusion rates depend on the size and molecular weight of the diffusing molecules relative to the scaffold's pore size, determined by their Stokes radii [33, 38, 50]. Small molecules, such as glucose, oxygen, and vitamin B12, with molecular weights below 1300 Da and Stokes radii under 1 nm, can easily diffuse through ionically crosslinked alginate microspheres. In contrast, larger molecules like myoglobin, albumin, and fibrinogen face restricted movement, particularly as alginate concentration, calcium levels, and gelation increase. Similarly, higher crosslinker concentrations reduce diffusion rates in glutaraldehyde crosslinked chitosan gels. In PEO hydrogels, larger molecules can diffuse more easily as polymer molecular weight and hydrolyzable links increase. For charged molecules, diffusion is not solely size-dependent [51, 52]. In alginate and other charged polymers, interactions between the molecule's charge and the negatively charged polymer chains significantly affect diffusion rates. The scaffold's application dictates its diffusion requirements and material selection. While restricting diffusion is necessary for controlled molecule release, enhancing nutrient and oxygen transport is critical for cell survival. Since cells typically reside within 100 μm of a capillary in vivo, diffusion suffices over this distance. For longer distances, additional transport mechanisms like angiogenesis are required.

7.3.3 Biological Properties

Hydrogels used in the body must support tissue growth and promote cellular functions like adhesion, proliferation, and differentiation while minimizing long-term inflammatory responses. Hydrogel-forming polymers are typically designed to be biocompatible, ensuring they do not harm surrounding tissues or the cells they deliver. Collagen and hyaluronic acid (HA), key components of the natural extracellular matrix (ECM), are commonly used, with minimal immunogenic risk when properly processed. Bovine-derived collagen and HA generally interact well with human tissue, provided there are no cross-species immune reactions. Polyethylene oxide (PEO) is FDA-approved for various medical applications, while P(PF-co-EG) shows minimal toxicity and low inflammatory response [53]. Chitosan, despite its chemotactic effect on neutrophils, is considered non-toxic. Alginate's immunogenicity was once attributed to its high M content, but recent studies suggest impurities as the primary cause. Purified alginate is largely immunologically inert, though commercial alginate still faces purity challenges. While many hydrogels are biocompatible, they often lack cell-adhesive properties. Most cells do not have receptors for hydrogel polymers, except for collagen, which naturally promotes adhesion. The hydrophilic nature of hydrogels also limits the diffusion of ECM proteins like laminin, fibronectin, and vitronectin to their surface. To address this, researchers have developed specific adhesive surfaces by covalently attaching ECM proteins or bioactive peptides to hydrogel polymers [54, 55]. One common strategy is the covalent binding of peptides interacting with cellular receptors. The tripeptide sequence arginine–glycine–aspartic acid (RGD), derived from ECM proteins such as collagen, fibronectin, laminin, and vitronectin, is widely used to enhance cell adhesion. RGD modifications have been applied to alginate and PEG to improve cell attachment. Other peptides, such as YIGSR (from laminin), REDV (from fibronectin), and IKVAV (from laminin), are also used for specific cell interactions. Additionally, whole proteins like fibronectin have been conjugated to polymers such as PVA to promote adhesion. These modifications help hydrogels create a bioactive surface, encouraging cell attachment and enhancing their functionality in tissue engineering applications [56]. Hydrogels can be modified to regulate cellular activities by incorporating and tethering growth factors. Similar to adhesion proteins and peptides, growth factors and peptides derived from them can be covalently linked to hydrogel polymers. For example, transforming growth factor-beta (TGF-β) was attached to PEG to promote extracellular matrix (ECM) production in smooth muscle cells. Similarly, alginate was modified with an oligopeptide derived from bone morphogenetic protein-2 (BMP-2) to stimulate osteoblast migration and scaffold calcification. Additionally, hydrogels can be loaded with various compounds to influence tissue development [57, 58].

7.4 Hydrogel Applications

Hydrogels serve diverse roles in tissue engineering, acting as space fillers, carriers of bioactive molecules, and 3D frameworks that organize cells and provide signals for tissue formation. As space-filling agents, hydrogels have various applications, including bulking, preventing adhesions, and functioning as biological "glue." They also deliver bioactive compounds for purposes such as encapsulating secretory cells and promoting angiogenesis. Additionally, hydrogel scaffolds are being used to develop a wide range of tissues, including smooth muscle, bone, and cartilage, and to facilitate cell transplantation.

7.4.1 *Scaffolds for Filling Spaces*

Space-filling hydrogels serve as bulking agents, bioadhesives, or anti-adhesive barriers, with their primary design requirements being the ability to maintain volume and structural stability for a set duration. These hydrogels are widely used in cosmetic and reconstructive surgery and treat conditions like vesicoureteral reflux and urinary incontinence [59, 60]. Additionally, they function as biological adhesives and help prevent post-operative adhesions. Materials such as collagen, chitosan, and alginate are commonly explored as general bulking agents. Studies show promising results using RGD-modified alginate scaffolds in rats, demonstrating significant tissue ingrowth, minimal encapsulation, and a negligible immune response [61]. Similarly, porous chitosan scaffolds implanted in mice showed limited encapsulation and a mild immune reaction, though tissue ingrowth was confined to the scaffold edges. Collagen scaffolds crosslinked with glutaraldehyde have been used as bulking agents for urinary incontinence, though their effectiveness varies, often requiring multiple injections due to collagen degradation by collagenase [62–64]. While glutaraldehyde reduces this degradation, it does not prevent it entirely, and vascular infiltration remains limited. A dextranomer/hyaluronic acid (HA) copolymer, used to treat vesicoureteral reflux, showed stability after a single injection, attributed to collagen deposition triggered by an inflammatory response [65]. Synthetic hydrogels, such as PEG and PVA, are effective anti-adhesive agents due to their non-adhesive properties. PEG has been applied to prevent arterial thickening and post-operative adhesions, with photocrosslinked PEG significantly reducing adhesions in rat and rabbit models. These PEG-based hydrogels typically resorb within five days. Another approach involves grafting PEG onto poly L-lysine (PLL), creating a copolymer (PLL-g-PEG) that adheres to tissue on one side and provides a non-adhesive surface on the other, although it forms a liquid rather than a gel at the application site [65–68]. In contrast, biological adhesives are designed to enhance wound healing and seal small openings that could leak fluids or air. Traditionally, fibrin glue has been used, but chitosan-based hydrogels and chitin derivatives are now being explored for this purpose. Photocrosslinked chitosan gels have successfully sealed pinholes in mice's trachea, aorta, and intestines, demonstrating in vitro safety. Overall, hydrogels offer versatile applications as space fillers, adhesion barriers, and bioadhesives, supporting tissue repair, preventing unwanted adhesions, and enhancing wound sealing in various medical contexts [69].

7.4.2 *Scaffolds for Bioactive Molecule Delivery*

Hydrogel scaffolds are increasingly used to encapsulate secretory cells and deliver bioactive compounds locally, distinguishing them from simple space-filling agents. While many drugs are systemically administered via oral or intravenous routes, this approach often leads to inefficient targeting due to enzymatic degradation and non-specific tissue absorption, necessitating high doses and risking systemic side effects. For instance, systemic administration of vascular endothelial growth factor (VEGF), which promotes localized angiogenesis, can inadvertently lead to tumor growth, plaque expansion, and unwanted tissue neovascularization [70–73]. Thus, scaffolds that allow controlled, site-specific drug release are highly desirable. Hydrogels effectively integrate and release proteins, particularly VEGF, which is incorporated into ionically crosslinked alginate and collagen sponges. VEGF release occurs via scaffold degradation or diffusion, and studies show enhanced bioactivity when VEGF is stabilized within alginate microspheres, promoting angiogenesis in vitro and in vivo. Similarly, heparin-alginate gels facilitate the sustained release of basic fibroblast growth factor (bFGF), another angiogenic protein. Bone morphogenetic proteins (BMPs) like BMP-2 are also delivered using hydrogel scaffolds to promote osteogenesis [74–77]. For example, BMP-2 incorporated into photocrosslinked PLA-PEG and PLA-DX-PEG systems induces bone growth as the polymer degrades. In vivo, these scaffolds only triggered bone formation when BMP-2 concentrations exceeded 0.5 mg. Other systems, such as porous hyaluronic acid scaffolds, also achieve sustained, active BMP-2 release. Beyond protein delivery, various hydrogel systems are used for drug delivery, including PEG bilayers, glutaraldehyde-crosslinked chitosan microspheres, thermosensitive PEG-PLLA gels, and degradable PEO-PLLA gels. Cell encapsulation within hydrogels offers a unique approach for sustained drug release, particularly in enzyme and hormone deficiencies. Encapsulated cells continuously produce therapeutic compounds in response to the body's needs, providing a long-term solution [78, 79].

Alginate, known for its non-degradability, mild gelling conditions, and ease of mixing with cells, is a popular choice for encapsulating primary cells like hepatocytes, adrenal cortical cells, pancreatic islets, and genetically modified cells. Common systems include ionically crosslinked alginate microcapsules coated with poly-L-lysine (PLL) or PEG. Encapsulated pancreatic islets have shown success in glucose-sensitive insulin release, facilitating xenotransplantation. Photocrosslinked PEG systems also yield similar results. However, challenges remain [80]. Diffusion limitations, particularly for oxygen, restrict capsule size and reduce cell viability at the core. Fibrotic encapsulation, caused by alginate impurities, hinders permeability and insulin release, leading to cell death. Strategies to mitigate this include additional PEG coatings and purifying alginate to prolong islet function. Additionally, hemoglobin immobilization within alginate microcapsules enhances oxygen transport, improving cell survival. Overall, hydrogel-based drug delivery systems, particularly for proteins and encapsulated cells, hold promise for treating diabetes and hormone or enzyme deficiencies. By enabling localized, controlled release and reducing systemic side effects, these scaffolds offer a targeted, efficient therapeutic approach [81, 82].

7.4.3 Scaffolds for Cell Delivery

Hydrogel scaffolds are three-dimensional, highly hydrated polymer networks that create an optimal environment for tissue development by supporting cell adhesion, proliferation, and differentiation. These scaffolds can transmit chemical cues through the incorporation of growth factors and mechanical signals by adjusting their mechanical properties. Current research focuses on designing tissues like cartilage, bone, muscle, fat, liver, and neurons using these scaffolds. Hydrogels resemble cartilage's structure, which consists of chondrocytes embedded in glycosaminoglycans (GAGs) and type II collagen [83]. This structural similarity makes hydrogels well-suited for cartilage engineering. Various chondrocyte-embedded hydrogel scaffolds have been developed and tested in vitro and in vivo, analyzing the effects of scaffold composition, growth factor delivery, and mechanical properties on chondrocyte behavior [84]. Stiffer scaffolds, such as photocrosslinked polyethylene oxide (PEO) and freeze-dried chitosan, exhibit high moduli (~500 kPa) and tend to keep chondrocytes in a proliferative state, reducing type II collagen production. Dual delivery of transforming growth factor-beta (TGF-β) and insulin-like growth factor (IGF-I) also maintained proliferation. Conversely, softer gels made from hyaluronic acid (HA) or HA combined with alginate promoted differentiation and type II collagen synthesis, with HA alone supporting both protein production and cell growth. While early cell proliferation is critical to ensure a sufficient population, the synthesis of GAGs and type II collagen ultimately determines successful cartilage formation [85–87]. Studies highlight key scaffold features that influence cartilage development. Alginate is one of the most commonly used hydrogels for in vivo cartilage engineering. It has been combined with chondrocytes and either injected or molded for implantation. Animal studies demonstrated viable chondrocytes and cartilage-like matrix production within four weeks, though the mechanical properties of the engineered cartilage were significantly lower than native tissue, with a compression modulus of 15% and hydraulic permeability of 20 times higher [88].

In human trials, alginate combined with autologous chondrocytes showed promise in treating urinary incontinence, with about 80% of patients improving after a single injection, outperforming collagen-based treatments that require multiple injections. Although new tissue formation was not directly observed in these trials, it was confirmed in animal studies. Hydrogel scaffolds are commonly used in non-load-bearing bone tissue engineering due to their minimal mechanical strength. However, their ability to be minimally invasively implanted into critical defects makes them valuable for encouraging bone regeneration in areas that might not heal otherwise. Both hyaluronic acid (HA) and alginate are frequently used in these applications [89–92]. For example, primary rat osteoblasts combined with PAG, a degradable alginate, were implanted in immunodeficient mice, resulting in bone mineralization within nine weeks, though this was limited to the outer portions of the implant due to nutrient transport limitations. Similarly, bone marrow stromal cells (BMSCs) seeded onto HA scaffolds led to bone repair in rat radial defects, with pre-treatment using basic fibroblast growth factor (bFGF) enhancing the outcome. In these cases, scaffolds primarily served as carriers for cell transport rather than actively guiding cell behavior. However, efforts have been made to engineer hydrogels with bioactive peptides to influence cell fate and promote bone formation. For instance, alginate scaffolds with covalently attached RGD peptides significantly increased bone formation compared to unmodified gels. Additionally, a BMP-2-derived peptide immobilized in alginate promoted ectopic bone growth, demonstrating that modifying hydrogels can enhance their ability to guide bone regeneration [93]. Hydrogels have also been explored for vascular smooth muscle engineering. Photocrosslinked PEG hydrogels with adhesion proteins, enzymatic degradation sites, and growth factors promoted greater collagen production and allowed cell migration, enhancing the development of functional vascular tissue when combined with external mechanical cues. Beyond bone and vascular tissue, hydrogels are being investigated for other tissues [94]. Peptide-modified alginate and collagen have shown potential in skeletal muscle engineering. Freeze-dried collagen sponges seeded with preadipocytes are being explored for adipose tissue formation, while collagen scaffolds have been used for large blood vessel engineering. Alginate hydrogels support hepatocyte function and liver-specific protein production and serve as scaffolds for Schwann cells in nerve grafts. As understanding of scaffold materials and factors influencing tissue growth advances, the ability to engineer functional tissues across the body continues to expand [95, 96].

7.5 Summary and Future Directions

A range of hydrogels, both natural and synthetic, are widely used or hold potential in tissue engineering. Natural hydrogels offer benefits like biocompatibility, cell-responsive degradation, and inherent bioactivity. However, they often have variable mechanical properties. Synthetic hydrogels can be precisely tailored in terms of structure and functionality but may require extensive purification due to the use of toxic chemicals in their production and the lack of biodegradability under physiological conditions. No single material can meet all design needs for every application, so various hydrogels will be used depending on specific requirements. A major challenge in tissue engineering is promoting vascularization to integrate engineered tissues with the host and supply nutrients. Hydrogels can facilitate localized delivery of angiogenic factors, such as VEGF, bFGF, EGF, and BMP, or endothelial cells, which form blood vessels. This targeted delivery encourages blood vessel formation within scaffolds, eventually connecting with the host's vasculature to create functional networks. Another strategy involves delivering genes encoding angiogenic proteins via plasmid DNA or co-transplanting endothelial cells with primary cells to promote rapid vascularization. Mechanical properties are crucial for hydrogels used in tissues like bone, muscle, and blood vessels, which exist in dynamic environments. Mechanical signals influence cellular behavior, gene expression, and tissue development. Designing hydrogels that transmit mechanical cues effectively and allow for controlled growth factor release in response to these signals could enhance tissue engineering in mechanically active environments.

The design of scaffolds plays a critical role in tissue engineering, bioactive molecule delivery, and space-filling applications, with the optimal design depending on the target tissue and its environment. For instance, scaffolds for bone or cartilage must account for load-bearing requirements, while the target site influences the delivery method for bioactive compounds. This creates a vast design space with numerous variables and interactions. To date, many materials have been chosen for specific properties, such as ease of cell incorporation, without fully considering other essential factors like mechanical strength or degradation behavior. Future advancements in material development will likely have a significant impact on tissue engineering. With an improved understanding of tissue growth, scaffolds must evolve to provide precise biological signals at appropriate times and locations. Additionally, the influence of external mechanical and electrical signals on synthetic tissue development will require further exploration. Innovative materials are already being developed to address these challenges. Hydrogels have been designed to control degradation rates, incorporate growth factors, and include cell-adhesion ligands to influence cell behavior. Various crosslinking techniques have improved biocompatibility and mechanical properties, while pre- and post-processing methods have been developed to regulate porosity, enhance diffusion, and enable gentle cell integration. These advancements are expected to enhance scaffold performance, supporting the creation of more functional and natural tissues.

References

1. Fisher JP, Mikos AG, Bronzino JD (1993) Tissue engineering. Science 260:1–583
2. Mooney DJ, Mikos AG (1999) Growing new organs. Sci Am 280:60–65
3. Putnam AJ, Mooney DJ (1996) Tissue engineering using synthetic extracellular matrices. Nat Med 2:824–826
4. Marler JJ, Upton J, Langer R, Vacanti JP (1998) Transplantation of cells in matrices for tissue regeneration. Adv Drug Deliv Rev 33:165–182
5. Niklason LE et al (1999) Functional arteries grown in vitro. Science 284:489–493
6. Pomahač B, Svensjö T, Yao F, Brown H, Eriksson E (1998) Tissue engineering of skin. Crit Rev Oral Biol Med 9:333–334
7. Oberpenning F, Meng J, Yoo JJ, Atala AD (1999) Novo reconstitution of a functional mammalian urinary bladder by tissue engineering. Nat Biotechnol 17:149–155
8. Vella F (1994) Molecular biology of the cell, 3rd edn by Alberts B, Bray D, Lewis J, Raff M, Roberts K, Watson JD (eds). Garland Publishing, New York and London, p 1361. Biochem Educ 22:164–164
9. Kim BS, Mooney DJ (1998) Development of biocompatible synthetic extracellular matrices for tissue engineering. Trends Biotechnol 16:224–230

10. Harris (1998) Open pore biodegradable matrices formed with gas foaming. J Biomed Mater Res. Wiley Online Library. https://onlinelibrary.wiley.com/doi/abs/10.1002/(SICI)1097-4636(19981205)42:3%3C396::AID-JBM7%3E3.0.CO%3B2-E
11. Thomson RC et al (1999) Guided tissue fabrication from periosteum using preformed biodegradable polymer scaffolds. Biomaterials 20:2007–2018
12. Babensee JE, Anderson JM, McIntire LV, Mikos AG (1998) Host response to tissue engineered devices. Adv Drug Deliv Rev 33:111–139
13. Řĺhová B (2000) Immunocompatibility and biocompatibility of cell delivery systems. Adv Drug Deliv Rev 42:65–80
14. LeRoux MA, Guilak F, Setton LA (1999) Compressive and shear properties of alginate gel: effects of sodium ions and alginate concentration. J Biomed Mater Res 47:46–53
15. Bromberg LE, Ron ES (1998) Temperature-responsive gels and thermogelling polymer matrices for protein and peptide delivery. Adv Drug Deliv Rev 31:197–221
16. Lee KY, Rowley JA, Eiselt P, Moy EM, Bouhadir KH, Mooney DJ (2000) Controlling mechanical and swelling properties of alginate hydrogels independently by cross-linker type and cross-linking density. Macromolecules 33:4291–4294. Scientific Research Publishing. https://www.scirp.org/reference/referencespapers?referenceid=973166
17. Cruise GM, Scharp DS, Hubbell JA (1998) Characterization of permeability and network structure of interfacially photopolymerized poly(ethylene glycol) diacrylate hydrogels. Biomaterials 19:1287–1294
18. Xiao X, Wu G, Zhou H, Qian K, Hu J (2017) Preparation and property evaluation of conductive hydrogel using poly (vinyl alcohol)/polyethylene glycol/graphene oxide for human electrocardiogram acquisition. Polymers (Basel) 9
19. Bryant SJ, Anseth KS (2001) The effects of scaffold thickness on tissue engineered cartilage in photocrosslinked poly(ethylene oxide) hydrogels. Biomaterials 22:619–626
20. Metters AT, Anseth KS, Bowman CN (2000) Fundamental studies of a novel, biodegradable PEG-b-PLA hydrogel. Polymer (Guildf) 41:3993–4004
21. Smidsrød O, Skjåk-Bræk G (1990) Alginate as immobilization matrix for cells. Trends Biotechnol 8:71–78
22. In vitro cytotoxicity and in vivo biocompatibility of poly(propylene fumarate-co-ethylene glycol) hydrogels. PubMed. https://pubmed.ncbi.nlm.nih.gov/10357132/
23. He S, Yaszemski MJ, Yasko AW, Engel PS, Mikos AG (2000) Injectable biodegradable polymer composites based on poly(propylene fumarate) crosslinked with poly(ethylene glycol)-dimethacrylate. Biomaterials 21:2389–2394
24. Lee CH, Singla A, Lee Y (2001) Biomedical applications of collagen. Int J Pharm 221:1–22
25. Chelu M, Moreno JMC, Musuc AM, Popa M (2024) Natural regenerative hydrogels for wound healing. Gels 10:547
26. Francis Suh JK, Matthew HWT (2000) Application of chitosan-based polysaccharide biomaterials in cartilage tissue engineering: a review. Biomaterials 21:2589–2598
27. Lee CR, Grodzinsky AJ, Spector M (2001) The effects of cross-linking of collagen-glycosaminoglycan scaffolds on compressive stiffness, chondrocyte-mediated contraction, proliferation and biosynthesis. Biomaterials 22:3145–3154
28. Schoof H, Apel J, Heschel I, Rau G (2001) Control of pore structure and size in freeze-dried collagen sponges. J Biomed Mater Res 58:352–357
29. Mensitieri M, Ambrosio L, Nicolais L, Bellini D, O'Regan M (1996) Viscoelastic properties modulation of a novel autocrosslinked hyaluronic acid polymer. J Mater Sci Mater Med 7:695–698
30. Borzacchiello A, Ambrosio L (2001) Network formation of low molecular weight hyaluronic acid derivatives. J Biomater Sci Polym Ed 12:307–316
31. Gamini A et al (2002) Structural investigations of cross-linked hyaluronan. Biomaterials 23:1161–1167
32. Fujiwara (2000) Gelation of hyaluronic acid through annealing. Polym Int. Wiley Online Library. https://scijournals.onlinelibrary.wiley.com/doi/abs/10.1002/1097-0126%28200012%2949%3A12%3C1604%3A%3AAID-PI558%3E3.0.CO%3B2-4

33. Singh G, Yadav P, Chanda A (2024) Development of biofidelic skin simulants based on fresh cadaveric skin tests. Eur Burn J 5:454–463
34. Singh G, Chanda A (2024) Biofidelic gallbladder tissue surrogates. Adv Mater Process Technol. https://doi.org/10.1080/2374068X.2023.2198835
35. Lim F, Moss RD (1981) Microencapsulation of living cells and tissues. J Pharm Sci 70:351–354
36. Singh G, Chanda A (2024) Development and biomechanical testing of artificial surrogates for vaginal tissue. Adv Mater Process Technol. https://doi.org/10.1080/2374068X.2023.2198837
37. Singh G, Chanda A (2022) Biomechanical modeling of progressive wound healing: a computational study. Biomed Eng Adv 4:100055
38. Singla R, Gupta S, Chanda A (2023) A computational fluid dynamics-based model for assessing rupture risk in cerebral arteries with varying aneurysm sizes. Math Comput Appl 28:90
39. Butler DL, Goldstein SA, Guilak F (2000) Functional tissue engineering: the role of biomechanics. J Biomech Eng 122:570–575
40. Chhikara K, Gupta S, Bose D, Kataria C, Chanda A (2023) Development and trial of a multipurpose customized orthosis for activities of daily living in patients with spinal cord injury. Prosthesis 5:467–479
41. Rothschild BM et al (2023) Design, manufacturing, and trial of a 3D printed customized finger splint for patients with rheumatoid arthritis. Rheumato 3:51–62
42. Chanda A, McClain S (2019) Mechanical modeling of healthy and diseased calcaneal fat pad surrogates. Biomimetics 4:1
43. Sikavitsas VI, Temenoff JS, Mikos AG (2001) Biomaterials and bone mechanotransduction. Biomaterials 22:2581–2593
44. Bryant SJ, Anseth KS (2002) Hydrogel properties influence ECM production by chondrocytes photoencapsulated in poly(ethylene glycol) hydrogels. J Biomed Mater Res 59:63–72
45. Chanda A, Ruchti T, Unnikrishnan V (2018) Computational modeling of wound suture: a review. IEEE Rev Biomed Eng 11:165–176
46. Stammen JA, Williams S, Ku DN, Guldberg RE (2001) Mechanical properties of a novel PVA hydrogel in shear and unconfined compression. Biomaterials 22:799–806
47. Saito N et al (2001) A biodegradable polymer as a cytokine delivery system for inducing bone formation. Nat Biotechnol 194(19):332–335
48. Gupta V, Singh G, Chanda A (2023) Development of hierarchical auxetic skin graft simulants with high expansion potential. Biomed Eng Adv 5:100087
49. Gupta V, Chanda A (2023) Auxetic incisions with alternating slit shapes: a promising technique for enhancing synthetic skin grafts expansion. Mater Res Express 10:075802
50. Lu S, Anseth KS (2000) Release behavior of high molecular weight solutes from poly(ethylene glycol)-based degradable networks. Macromolecules 33:2509–2515
51. Tanaka H, Matsumura M, Veliky IA (1984) Diffusion characteristics of substrates in Ca-alginate gel beads. Biotechnol Bioeng 26:53–58
52. Transport characterization of hydrogel matrices for cell encapsulation. PubMed. https://pubmed.ncbi.nlm.nih.gov/18626985/
53. Ueno H, Mori T, Fujinaga T (2001) Topical formulations and wound healing applications of chitosan. Adv Drug Deliv Rev 52:105–115
54. Klöck G et al (1997) Biocompatibility of mannuronic acid-rich alginates. Biomaterials 18:707–713
55. Yadav P, Singh G, Gupta S, Chanda A (2025) Biomechanical characterization of cadaveric thigh skin for development of biofidelic simulants. Clin Biomech 129:106650
56. Zhang WJ, Laue C, Hyder A, Schrezenmeir J (2001) Purity of alginate affects the viability and fibrotic overgrowth of encapsulated porcine islet xenografts. Transplant Proc 33:3517–3519
57. Mann BK, Schmedlen RH, West JL (2001) Tethered-TGF-beta increases extracellular matrix production of vascular smooth muscle cells. Biomaterials 22:439–444
58. Majumdar P, Singh G, Chanda A (2024) Development and biomechanical testing of full-scale human brain simulant. J Eng Res. https://doi.org/10.1016/J.JER.2024.02.016
59. Pediatric urinary tract infection and reflux. PubMed. https://pubmed.ncbi.nlm.nih.gov/10193590/

60. Seibold J et al (2011) Long-term results after endoscopic VUR-treatment using dextranomer/hyaluronic acid copolymer—5-year experience in a single-center. Cent Eur J Urol 64:84
61. In vivo characterization of a porous hydrogel material for use as a tissue bulking agent. PubMed. https://pubmed.ncbi.nlm.nih.gov/11553888/
62. Zhao X, Kato K, Fukumoto Y, Nakamae K (2001) Synthesis of bioadhesive hydrogels from chitin derivatives. Int J Adhes Adhes 21:227–232
63. Chanda A, Callaway C (2018) Tissue anisotropy modeling using soft composite materials. Appl Bionics Biomech 2018:4838157
64. Yadav P et al (2025) Gelatin multiwalled carbon nanotube composite 3D printed semi biological mesh for abdominal hernia treatment. Chem Asian J 20:e202401136
65. West JL, Hubbell JA (1996) Separation of the arterial wall from blood contact using hydrogel barriers reduces intimal thickening after balloon injury in the rat: the roles of medial and luminal factors in arterial healing. Proc Natl Acad Sci 93:13188–13193
66. Hill-West JL, Chowdhury SM, Slepian MJ, Hubbell JA (1994) Inhibition of thrombosis and intimal thickening by in situ photopolymerization of thin hydrogel barriers. Proc Natl Acad Sci 91:5967–5971
67. Ellahi A, Gupta S, Bose D, Chanda A (2025) A high-fidelity biomechanical modeling framework for injury prediction during frontal car crash. Comput Methods Biomech Biomed Engin 28:13–24
68. Gupta V, Singh G, Chanda A (2023) Modeling of metamaterial based incision patterns for generating high expansions in skin grafts. Clin Biomech 110:106118
69. Prevention of postoperative adhesions in the rat by in situ photopolymerization of bioresorbable hydrogel barriers. PubMed. https://pubmed.ncbi.nlm.nih.gov/8272310/
70. Simons M et al (2000) Clinical trials in coronary angiogenesis: issues, problems, consensus: an expert panel summary. Circulation 102
71. Epstein SE, Fuchs S, Zhou YF, Baffour R, Kornowski R (2001) Therapeutic interventions for enhancing collateral development by administration of growth factors: basic principles, early results and potential hazards. Cardiovasc Res 49:532–542
72. Gupta V, Singla R, Chanda A (2023) Development and Characterization of Novel Anisotropic Skin Graft Simulants. Dermato 3:114–130
73. Singh G, Chanda A (2024) Finite element modeling of diabetic foot: a state-of-the-art review. Eng Res Express 6:012507
74. Valentini RF, Kim HD (2002) Retention and activity of BMP-2 in hyaluronic acid-based scaffolds in vitro. J Biomed Mater Res 59:573–584
75. Singh G, Gupta V, Chanda A (2022) Artificial skin with varying biomechanical properties. Mater Today Proc 62:3162–3166
76. Gupta V, Gupta S, Chanda A (2023) Development of an ultra-low-cost planar biaxial tester for soft tissue characterization. Biomed Phys Eng Express 9:025011
77. Yadav P, Kamboj M, Das B (2024) Application of nanotechnology in antimicrobial coating on surgical instruments. Appl Nanotechnol Biomed Eng 150–168. https://doi.org/10.1201/978 1003432661-9
78. An Y, Hubbell JA (2000) Intraarterial protein delivery via intimally-adherent bilayer hydrogels. J Control Release 64:205–215
79. Gupta V, Singh G, Chanda A, Chanda A (2021) Expansion potential of skin grafts with novel I-shaped auxetic incisions. Biomed Phys Eng Express 8:015016
80. Cruise GM et al (1999) In vitro and in vivo performance of porcine islets encapsulated in interfacially photopolymerized poly(ethylene glycol) diacrylate membranes. Cell Transplant 8:293–306
81. Sawhney AS, Pathak CP, Hubbell JA (1993) Interfacial photopolymerization of poly(ethylene glycol)-based hydrogels upon alginate-poly(l-lysine) microcapsules for enhanced biocompatibility. Biomaterials 14:1008–1016
82. Singh G, Gupta V, Chanda A (2022) Mechanical characterization of rotating triangle shaped auxetic skin graft simulants. Facta Univ Ser Mech Eng

83. Grigolo B et al (2002) Evidence for redifferentiation of human chondrocytes grown on a hyaluronan-based biomaterial (HYAff 11): molecular, immunohistochemical and ultrastructural analysis. Biomaterials 23:1187–1195
84. Atala A, Kim W, Paige KT, Vacanti CA, Retik AB (1994) Endoscopic treatment of vesicoureteral reflux with a chondrocyte-alginate suspension. J Urol 152:641–643
85. Lisignoli G et al (2002) Osteogenesis of large segmental radius defects enhanced by basic fibroblast growth factor activated bone marrow stromal cells grown on non-woven hyaluronic acid-based polymer scaffold. Biomaterials 23:1043–1051
86. Chanda A, Gupta V, Gupta S (2024) Development and mechanical testing of auxetic incisions on human cadaveric skin, pp 89–99. https://doi.org/10.1007/978-981-97-4383-4_7
87. Chanda A (2018) Biomechanical modeling of human skin tissue surrogates. Biomimetics 3
88. Vandenburgh HH, Karlisch P, Farr L (1988) Maintenance of highly contractile tissue-cultured avian skeletal myotubes in collagen gel. In Vitro Cell Dev Biol 24:166–174
89. Vandenburgh HH, Hatfaludy S, Karlisch P, Shansky J (1989) Skeletal muscle growth is stimulated by intermittent stretch-relaxation in tissue culture. Am J Physiol 256
90. Verma S, Singh G, Chanda A (2024) Development of a computational framework for determination of detrimental vibrations on the human spine segments. Multiscale Sci Eng 61(6):48–56
91. Gupta V, Chanda A (2024) Mechanical characterization of alternating slit, I-shaped and rotating triangle based auxetic skin graft phantoms. Mech Adv Mater Struct. https://doi.org/10.1080/15376494.2023.2250782
92. Verma S, Chanda A (2024) State-of-the-art of finite element modelling of the human spine to study the impact of vibrations: a review. Int J Comput Methods Eng Sci Mech 25:225–247
93. Okano T, Matsuda T (1998) Tissue engineered skeletal muscle: Preparation of highly dense, highly oriented hybrid muscular tissues. Cell Transplant 7:71–82
94. Rowley JA, Mooney DJ (2002) Alginate type and RGD density control myoblast phenotype. J Biomed Mater Res 60:217–223
95. Yang J et al (2001) Hepatocyte-specific porous polymer-scaffolds of alginate/galactosylated chitosan sponge for liver-tissue engineering. Biotechnol Lett 23:1385–1389
96. Chanda A, Gupta S (2025) Healthcare entrepreneurship and management. Routledge, Taylor & Francis Group

Chapter 8
Nanotechnology-Based Artificial Tissues

8.1 Introduction

With the rise in age-related and lifestyle-induced diseases, the demand for tissue-engineered constructs has increased significantly. These constructs offer a promising alternative to conventional organ transplantation. Nanotechnology has played a pivotal role in advancing this field, particularly through the use of nanoparticles and nanomaterials, which have transformed both medical imaging and implant development. By integrating nanotechnology into medicine, there's great potential to enhance human health and quality of life. For instance, nanoparticles can help minimize inflammation, combat infection, and, when used in combination, accelerate early tissue formation, thereby extending the functional lifespan of implants. Nanotechnology has shown direct relevance in addressing major medical challenges such as cancer, cardiovascular diseases, and congenital disorders. A key focus in clinical nanomedicine is utilizing nanoscale materials for stem cell therapy and cancer treatment. A notable example is the successful implantation of the world's first synthetic trachea, constructed from a nanocomposite polymer and seeded with a patient's own stem cells, for the treatment of airway cancer. This success, along with the limitations of older microscale technologies, underscores nanotechnology's crucial role in overcoming current medical challenges. Moving forward, nanotechnology is expected to drive the development of biomimetic nano-biomaterials that can match or even surpass the functions of natural tissues and organs. This chapter discusses the advantages of employing nanotechnology, either on its own or in combination with other materials, to develop scaffolds and artificial organs for tissue engineering. It also explores how cells respond to biomaterials at the nanoscale and examines the design and optimization of unique nanoscale surface features for various biomedical applications. Furthermore, it highlights the evolving trends in nanotechnology over time [1–3].

A. Chanda and D. Sharma, *Handbook of Artificial Tissues, Biofabrication and Bioprinting, Volume I*, Biomedical Materials for Multi-functional Applications,
https://doi.org/10.1007/978-981-92-1307-8_8

8.2 Nanoparticles and Their Role in Developing Nanomaterials

Nanoparticles (NPs) are typically defined as particles ranging in size from 1 to 100 nm. Due to their diverse applications and potential impact across multiple fields, extensive research has recently been devoted to exploring NPs. Unlike their bulk counterparts, materials at the nanoscale often display unique and enhanced properties. Incorporating NPs into other materials leads to the formation of innovative nanocomposites that possess distinctive characteristics. In tissue engineering and regenerative medicine, nanoparticles play a key role in several areas: enhancing in vitro and in vivo imaging techniques, enabling the tracking of cellular and tissue development and their in-body behavior, facilitating targeted drug delivery and therapeutic cell guidance, aiding in the fabrication of nanocomposite scaffolds for cells or tissues, offering antimicrobial benefits and promoting wound healing, and providing electroconductive functions (see Fig. 8.1). A wide variety of nanoparticles have shown substantial potential in biological applications following their evaluation in diverse contexts. The specific properties of each type of NP has demonstrated promising opportunities for the development of artificial organs, as illustrated by the following examples.

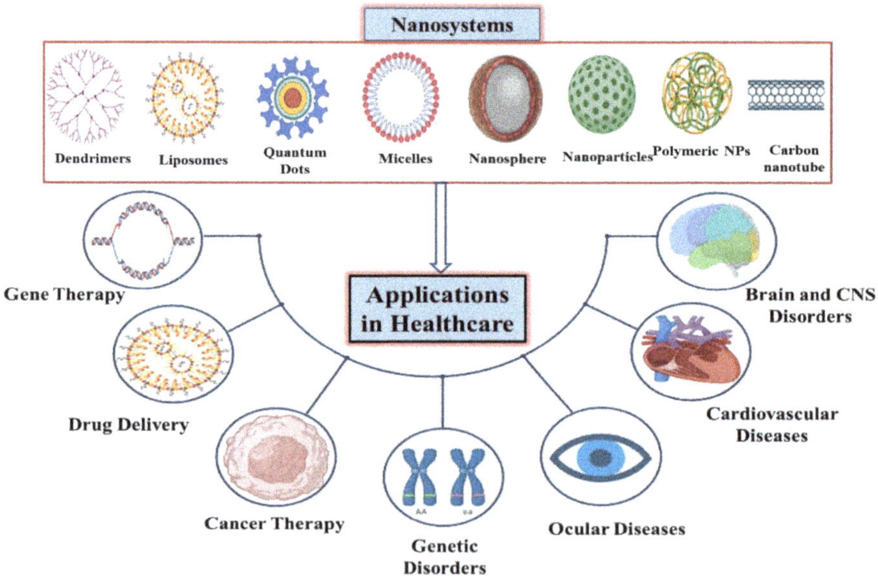

Fig. 8.1 Overview of nanosystems utilization across various allied healthcare fields. Figure reproduced under license CC BY 4.0 [4] (https://creativecommons.org/licenses/by/4.0/)

8.2.1 Quantum Dots (QD)

Photostability is crucial for applications involving fluorescence. Among available techniques, fluorescence-based methods have proven to be both effective and practical for real-time detection. Quantum dots (QDs), in particular, offer excellent long-term photostability. Unlike organic fluorophores, QDs are highly resistant to photobleaching and can maintain consistent fluorescence even after numerous exposures [5–7]. However, concerns remain primarily regarding the composition of QDs. Efforts have been made to reduce toxicity by developing thinner or less harmful coatings. For example, pathological studies in rats injected with amphiphilic polymer (amp)-coated CdSe-ZnS QDs indicated minimal or negligible toxicity. Moreover, fluorescence signals from these QDs were retained for over two years [8, 9]. The hydrodynamic diameter (HD) of QDs significantly influences their excretion pathways. QDs with diameters below 5.5 nm were found to be rapidly and efficiently eliminated via urine, while those exceeding 15 nm may face barriers to renal clearance. Due to their unique characteristics, QDs enable in vivo tracking of various cell types [10, 11]. Their ability to emit infrared or near-infrared light also makes them highly effective for imaging deep tissues and cells. Currently, four main strategies exist for labeling cells with QDs: internalization of QDs by cells; attachment of QDs to cell surface proteins using peptide or antibody conjugates; direct cellular entry through conjugation with amphipathic peptides; and delivery via liposomes or micelles [12]. These labeling methods are actively being applied in research to observe the proliferation, differentiation, and migration of key cell types, such as mesenchymal stem cells (MSCs), within organs. In a study involving rabbits with osteochondral defects, MSCs labeled with anti-mortalin-QDs showed evidence of tissue integration and regeneration. These labeled cells also exhibited persistent fluorescence signals for at least 26 weeks during healing [13, 14]. Similarly, Qdot655-labeled human MSCs seeded on fibrin-based biological sutures and implanted into rat hearts were tracked for up to eight weeks post-implantation, with the QDs still present and eliciting a reduced fibrotic response. Additionally, QDs enable the simultaneous identification of multiple fluorescence colors.

8.2.2 Magnetic Nanoparticles (MNPs)

Magnetic nanoparticles (MNPs), typically composed of magnetic elements such as iron, nickel, cobalt, or their oxides, can be directed using external magnetic fields [15, 16]. Among them, iron oxide nanoparticles have drawn significant biomedical interest, particularly since they have received approval from the US Food and Drug Administration (FDA) [17]. These nanoparticles are known for their biocompatibility, non-toxicity, and ease of synthesis. The two main forms of iron oxide used are Fe_3O_4 (magnetite) and γ-Fe_2O_3 (maghemite). MNPs have been developed for various medical applications, including magnetic nanoparticle hyperthermia, as well as targeted drug delivery systems and contrast agents for magnetic resonance imaging (MRI), with potential as innovative cancer therapies. A recent study using superparamagnetic iron oxide (SPIO) nanoparticles demonstrated their utility as long-term cell tracking tools through multimodal imaging techniques such as MRI and X-ray microcomputed tomography (μCT). This was shown in engineered tissues seeded with muscle-derived progenitor cells and implanted into a rat's heart [18–20]. The results support the feasibility of non-invasive, long-term tracking—lasting up to one year in both in vivo and ex vivo conditions. Additional histological analysis confirmed that the transplanted cells retained the nanoparticles without releasing them or being phagocytosed by macrophages. Another notable example of in vivo MNP-based therapy involved a magnetic bifunctional cell engager (MagBICE). This platform was conjugated with two distinct antibodies—anti-CD45 and anti-CD34—enabling the connection of therapeutic bone marrow mesenchymal stem cells to injured cardiomyocytes. This interaction promoted angiogenesis and cardiomyogenesis, indicating the potential of MagBICE for inducing cell-mediated repair [21]. Such advances could contribute to the creation of a targeted cell therapy platform.

8.2.3 Polyhedral Oligomeric Silesquioxane (POSS)

Polyhedral oligomeric silsesquioxane (POSS) is an organosilicon compound with a cage-like structure that can adopt various geometries such as cubic, hexagonal, decagonal, or dodecagonal prisms. Its three-dimensional nanoscale framework and the ability to modify functional groups in all three dimensions make POSS a highly versatile building block for engineering nanocomposites. The silica-based core of POSS imparts rigidity and thermal resistance to polymeric materials, enhancing both mechanical and thermal performance compared to traditional materials. Another key feature of POSS-based materials is their biocompatibility. For instance, stents coated with POSS-PCU demonstrated increased adhesion of endothelial progenitor cells relative to control groups, and POSS-integrated poly(ester urethane) (PEU) supported the proliferation of mouse embryonic stem cells at levels similar to those cultured on gelatin. Due to these advantageous properties, POSS nanocomposites have been developed for various biomedical applications, including hydrogels, dental materials, polycaprolactone-based composites, and polyurethane-based systems [22–25]. POSS has also been incorporated into biodegradable linear thermoplastic polyurethanes composed of poly(ε-caprolactone) (PCL) and polyethylene glycol (PEG), using a surface passivation strategy that offers resistance to enzymatic and hydrolytic degradation for up to 22 days [26]. After the initial degradation phase, wavelength-dispersive X-ray spectrometry (WDS) confirmed that covalently attached POSS groups formed a nearly continuous protective layer. This layer shielded PCL's ester bonds from enzymatic attack, effectively halting further degradation. One notable nanocomposite, POSS-poly(carbonateurea)urethane (POSS-PCU), has been utilized in the fabrication of artificial organs such as vascular grafts, heart valves, lacrimal ducts, and artificial ears. In 2011, POSS-PCU was used to

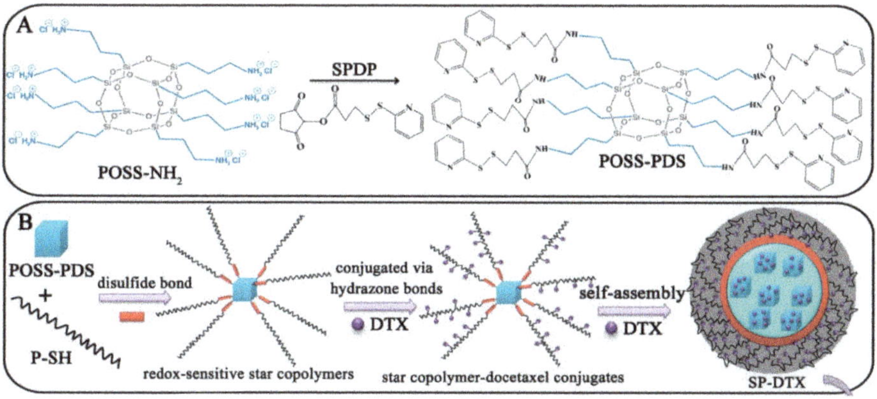

Fig. 8.2 **a** Synthetic route for obtaining pyridyldisulfanyl-modified polyhedral oligomeric silsesquioxane (POSS–PDS). **b** Development of SP-DTX nanoparticles via the self-assembly of amphiphilic star-shaped POSS-derived conjugates. Figure reproduced under license CC BY 4.0 [31] (https://creativecommons.org/licenses/by/4.0/)

develop the first synthetic trachea for clinical application. This scaffold, seeded with the patient's own stem cells and mimicking the extracellular matrix, was successfully implanted, promoting wound healing and showing potential for improved mechanical integrity and biocompatibility in long-term surgical implants. The material also supported graft remodeling and new blood vessel formation, underscoring the multifaceted advantages of incorporating POSS into biomedical devices [27–30] (see Fig. 8.2).

8.2.4 Silver Nanoparticles (AgNPs)

Silver nanoparticles (AgNPs) have gained considerable attention for their biological applications, especially due to their antimicrobial effects and selective toxicity toward microorganisms, which have raised concerns regarding their broader impact on human health and the environment. AgNPs have shown strong antimicrobial activity against a wide range of pathogens, including viruses, fungi, and multidrug-resistant bacteria. When incorporated into other materials, AgNPs can enhance their antibacterial effectiveness. For example, embedding AgNPs into zeolite, a porous, crystalline hydrated sodium aluminum silicate, resulted in an Ag/zeolite composite with antibacterial effects against both gram-positive and gram-negative bacteria, such as *Staphylococcus aureus*, methicillin-resistant *S. aureus*, *Escherichia coli*, and *Shigella dysenteriae* [32]. Silver-based wound dressings, which are commercially available, are commonly used for treating infections and aiding skin regeneration. However, their clinical use remains controversial due to the potential risks associated with prolonged silver exposure, such as argyria. Studies assessing AgNP cytotoxicity have shown that exposure to various concentrations (12.5–200 μg/mL) in human and mammalian cells may increase oxidative stress, activate heat shock proteins, damage DNA, and trigger the production of reactive oxygen species (ROS) [33]. Consequently, the total silver content plays a pivotal role in determining the antibacterial effectiveness of the product. Additional key factors that influence the antibacterial performance of AgNP-containing materials include the nanoparticles' dispersion, their chemical and physical structures, and moisture absorption [34]. In other words, for an antibacterial agent to be effective, there must be a detailed evaluation of the distribution of AgNPs and their ability to release the correct dosage in the appropriate form within a suitable timeframe. Moreover, optimizing silver-composite materials requires a comprehensive understanding of their antimicrobial mechanisms and the kinetics of silver release [35–38].

8.2.5 Carbon Nanomaterials: Graphene-Based and Carbon Nanotube

Conductive carbon nanomaterials have been extensively studied since the discovery of single-walled carbon nanotubes (SWCNTs) by Iijima in 1991 [39, 40]. Graphene, carbon nanotubes (CNTs), and other carbon-based materials have drawn significant attention due to their exceptional electrical and mechanical properties, lightweight nature, and high conductivity. In 1999, it was reported that an electrochemical actuator utilizing SWCNTs could exhibit actuation behavior in an electrolyte environment [41]. Recently, the integration of carbon nanomaterials into electrochemical devices has become increasingly relevant in medical and scientific fields. Particularly, ionic polymer-metal composite (IPMC) actuators have received notable interest because of their large strain response at low voltage and ability to function in air. These actuators typically consist of an ion-conductive membrane sandwiched between two electron-conductive metal electrodes. When voltage is applied, ion migration causes expansion and contraction in the electrodes, resulting in bending motion. The performance of these actuators largely depends on the electrochemical and electromechanical properties of the electrode layer. Improving the design of this layer can significantly enhance actuator performance. By combining the advantages of graphene and CNTs, new three-dimensional (3D) graphene/CNT films have shown remarkable improvements in mechanical strength, electrochemical capacity, and conductivity. Consequently, IPMC actuators utilizing these 3D electrodes demonstrated promising durability and responsive actuation behavior. Electro-responsive behavior has also been observed in polymer-based implants designed for on-demand drug release. A graphene-based hydrogel hybrid electroactive scaffold was able to modulate drug delivery through ON/OFF cycles of low-voltage stimulation, showing effective performance in in vivo tests without inducing unwanted heat. Nonetheless, because cellular responses are highly sensitive to nanoparticle characteristics such as size, shape, solubility, and concentration, the potential toxicity of graphene and CNTs warrants careful investigation. Additional in vitro and in vivo studies are necessary to fully understand their biocompatibility and safety for medical use [42–45]. Each nanoparticle (NP) type offers unique properties and, in some cases, overlapping applications. These functionalities can be harnessed to enhance material performance, potentially enabling the creation of "smart artificial organs" tailored to clinical needs. For instance, magnetic nanoparticles (MNPs) can be used to aid in drug delivery, track implant position, and mediate cell therapy for visual impairment. Quantum dots (QDs) are useful for real-time tracking of cells and implants and may also support drug delivery. Polyhedral oligomeric silsesquioxane (POSS) can enhance mechanical integrity, slow degradation, or provide non-degradable scaffold options. Silver nanoparticles (AgNPs), when properly dosed, can prevent infection and support wound healing. Carbon nanomaterials have shown potential for use in electroactive actuators, electro-responsive drug delivery systems, and even artificial muscle applications. In one example, a graphene-POSS modified poly(caprolactone-based urea-urethane) (PCL) hybrid nanocomposite was developed, combining the extended degradation time contributed by POSS with the electrical conductivity of graphene to produce superior mechanical performance [46]. This integrated strategy could lead to the development of smart artificial organs that leverage the synergistic benefits of multiple NPs for therapeutic outcomes. However, the risk of NP accumulation in the body and their potential interactions with cellular proteins cannot be overlooked. A key challenge in this field remains the comprehensive understanding of NP toxicity and the need to modify or optimize nanoparticles to improve their safety and compatibility for biomedical applications [47–50].

8.3 Surface Modifications of Materials for Improved Biological Responses

Polyurethanes (PUs) and their composites have been subjected to various surface modifications to improve their compatibility with the biological environments they interact with. Multiple strategies have been explored, ranging from multilayered approaches like anodization, sandblasting, laser radiation, acid-etching, and methods such as plasma spraying (see Fig. 8.3). These modifications aim to mimic the diverse surface features that naturally promote typical cellular behaviors. However, achieving precise control over characteristics like nanotopography, surface uniformity, and the specific chemical functionality of deposited materials remains difficult, even with recent technological advances. Consequently, the biological responses to these synthetic surfaces can only be validated through in vitro and in vivo testing, as accurately predicting them remains a significant challenge.

Designing a surface at the molecular level that can reliably guide surrounding biological activity continues to be a complex issue, with many concepts proving ineffective despite initial promise. Terms such as "biocompatible," "anti-thrombogenic," and "non-fouling" have been commonly used to describe the ideal properties of

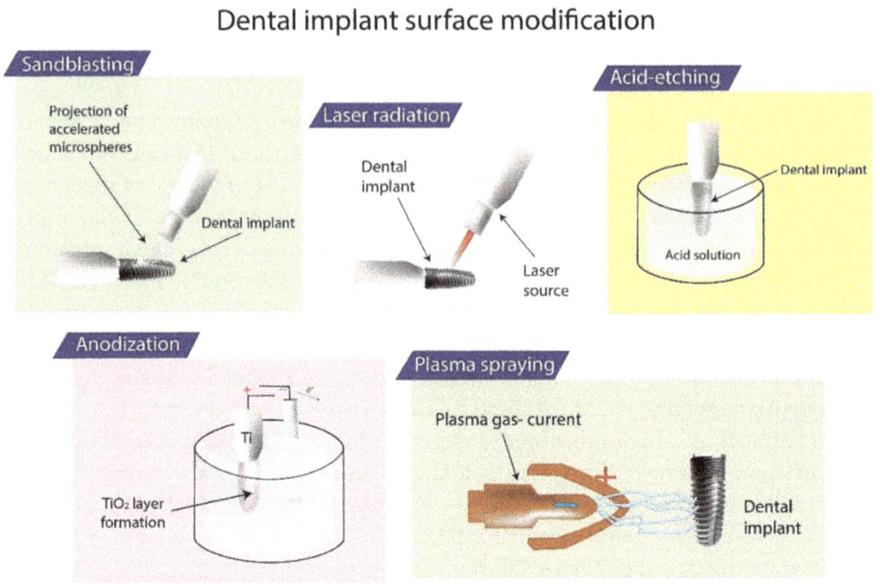

Fig. 8.3 Surface modifications in dental implants for improved biological responses. Figure reproduced under license CC BY 4.0 [51] (https://creativecommons.org/licenses/by/4.0/)

implantable materials. However, a closer examination of the body's response to implants often reveals that these terms are frequently misapplied, underscoring the critical role surface characteristics play in determining whether a device is ultimately "accepted" or "rejected" by the body.

- ***The Foreign Body Reaction and Biological Response***

The initial phase of the biological response to a synthetic surface involves the adsorption of proteins and water. Protein adhesion is largely influenced by the surface's hydrophilicity and chemical composition. Due to the non-specific nature of protein adsorption, both native and denatured proteins can bind to the surface, potentially contributing to the foreign body reaction. As part of the Vroman effect, initially adsorbed, less stable proteins are gradually displaced by proteins with a higher affinity for the surface. Cells such as macrophages, leukocytes, and platelets recognize these adsorbed proteins and initiate pro-inflammatory signaling pathways, which can ultimately lead to fibrosis, thrombosis, and chronic inflammation [52]. The electrostatic forces exerted by the chemical groups on the material's surface primarily determine which types of cells will colonize vascular implants. In the days immediately following implantation, neutrophils migrate to the site as part of the acute inflammatory response and release chemotactic agents that attract macrophages, which then work to eliminate the foreign material. Subsequently, tissue formation begins, involving blood vessels and plasma cells. If the surface properties of the material deviate significantly from those of native tissue, T-helper cells may trigger a prolonged inflammatory response. This typically involves the presence of foreign body giant cells and multinucleated macrophages, with their appearance depending on the mechanical properties of the implanted material. Additionally, blood flow in veins can introduce components that contribute to thrombosis during inflammation [53]. Surface modification strategies aim to influence the interactions between the synthetic material and the biological environment, thereby mitigating adverse responses like clot formation and foreign body reactions. Although a material may possess excellent bulk mechanical properties, this does not ensure that its surface is "biocompatible" or "anti-thrombogenic." For example, while unmodified PUs exhibit suitable mechanical performance for blood-contacting applications, currently available variants are unable to completely prevent thrombus formation. To address this, surface chemistry and properties can be tailored independently of the material's bulk traits. Because each material possesses distinct attributes, such as surface charge, designing a universal polymer for all biological environments is impractical. Therefore, the specific application and implantation site must be carefully considered. As a result, depending on the clinical context, terms such as thromboresistance, osseointegration, biodegradation, or non-fouling may be more appropriate than the generalized term "biocompatibility" to describe the desired surface behavior and to ensure long-term function and patency [54–57].

- ***Biomolecule Immobilization on the Material Surface***

As the initial point of contact with the body, surface chemistry plays a pivotal role in eliciting biological responses. Researchers now recognize the complexity of the biological environment, composed of various signals, and have explored multiple strategies to improve hemocompatibility, particularly for vascular prostheses. One widely studied approach involves pre-coating synthetic surfaces with endothelial cells to mimic native vascular linings. However, these pre-implantation strategies often lack long-term stability. Over the past two decades, pre-endothelialization and in situ endothelialization have dominated vascular graft research [58]. With advancements in surface engineering, attention has shifted toward developing composite materials that integrate biomolecule immobilization, surface functionalization, and desirable bulk mechanical properties. Commonly used agents include collagen, heparin, CD-34 antibodies, and sirolimus. Biomolecules, due to their inherent flexibility and specific recognition sites, enhance cellular interactions. Frequently used molecules such as heparin, RGD peptides, PEG, phospholipids, and antibodies aim to minimize non-specific adhesion, extend thrombin clotting time, and reduce surface hydrophobicity, thereby improving the compatibility of blood-contacting devices. Covalent attachment methods, like carbodiimide chemistry, are commonly used for binding peptides such as RGD to polyurethane (PU) or polyethylene (PE) surfaces. However, this method can lead to deactivation of reactive groups, a problem often addressed by protecting amines or using solvents like acetone or dichloromethane, though complete removal of toxic solvents before implantation is critical. Various techniques, including copolymerization, side-chain grafting, alkaline hydrolysis, and plasma treatment, have been employed to functionalize polymer surfaces. The RGD sequence, a minimal cell-binding domain from fibronectin, supports cell adhesion and accelerates endothelialization. Heparin maintains its anticoagulant properties when immobilized, promoting endothelial cell activity on grafts like ePTFE, though long-term outcomes have not surpassed standard PTFE after five years [59]. PEG, known for its protein-repellent properties, is used to reduce cell adhesion but suffers from instability due to oxidative degradation and inconsistent surface coverage. Phospholipids show excellent resistance to protein and bacterial adhesion. Grafting phospholipids onto PU with cerium-based initiators initially inhibits adhesion, but platelet accumulation occurs after 24 h. Zwitterionic groups like sulfobetaine further reduce protein adsorption but have yet to ensure long-term patency [60]. Antibodies offer high specificity but are costly and may lack selectivity due to shared receptors among cell types; numerous surface modification methods have been developed to immobilize biomolecules onto synthetic materials to improve biocompatibility. However, despite promising short-term results, achieving long-term functionality and patency remains a major challenge [60–63].

8.3.1 Surface Modification of Materials

These include methods that modify existing surface chemical groups through the use of reactive chemical solutions, and those that utilize plasma discharge to introduce new reactive species. Another distinct approach involves altering the polymer chains during synthesis. While this method also changes the surface chemistry, it simultaneously affects the material's bulk mechanical properties and degradation behavior.

- ***Surface Chemical Group Modification***

Heparin's anticoagulant properties are largely attributed to its negatively charged sulfonate groups, which have been shown to reduce cell adhesion [64, 65]. In one study, researchers introduced sulfonate groups into the hard segments of the polymer during synthesis by using diamino disulfonic acid as a chain extender, thereby modifying the polymer's terminal groups [62]. Although this approach increased sulfonate content and extended thrombin clotting time, the surface exhibited stronger fibrinogen adsorption compared to unmodified polyurethanes. Since fibrinogen is a key precursor in clot formation, this raised concerns about thrombogenicity. Another method involved generating surface radicals via Argon plasma treatment, followed by the grafting of a sulfoxy-terminated methacrylate compound to introduce sulfonate groups. Unlike UV-activated methods, this approach resulted in reduced thrombogenicity and hemolysis. The enhanced hydrophobicity associated with UV treatment may have facilitated protein adsorption that compromises erythrocyte membranes. In this plasma-based technique, slight reductions in protein adhesion and prothrombin clotting times were observed relative to control surfaces [66]. End-group modification presents another route for adding surface functionality, targeting terminal chemical groups such as isocyanates found in the hard segments of polyurethanes. Each modified end group must be individually assessed for cytotoxicity. One study utilized dimethylolpropionic acid to covalently attach hyaluronic acid to a carboxyl-functionalized polyurethane surface. Compared to control samples, the hyaluronic acid-modified surfaces showed improved hydrophilicity and significantly extended prothrombin clotting times. Additionally, cell adhesion was enhanced, in contrast to untreated PU and amine-terminated controls, which were reportedly cytotoxic. However, despite these promising short-term improvements, long-term patency has yet to be achieved [67].

- ***Surface Treatment by Deposition***

Over the last two decades, plasma polymerization has been widely employed for modifying material surfaces due to its efficiency and speed as a coating technique [68]. However, challenges persist. The process involves the introduction of vaporized radical species and the cleavage of homolytic bonds, which can lead to uneven surface coverage, inconsistent film thickness, and non-uniform coatings. These limitations arise from various side reactions and a general lack of selectivity. Therefore, it is essential to report the specific reaction conditions and provide detailed surface analysis when using plasma treatments. Studies have shown that perfluorocarbon functionalities on the surface of vascular grafts can facilitate protein binding [69]. While perfluorocarbons are considered "non-stick" in contexts like textiles, pipelines, and construction materials, their behavior in aqueous environments—such as the human body—is different. In water, the Hamaker constant changes substantially, making protein adsorption energetically favorable. This leads many proteins to undergo conformational changes upon binding. However, the structural changes in adhesive glycoproteins make it more difficult for endothelial cells and platelets to adhere to surfaces like PTFE, resulting in reduced cell adhesion. Each surface modification method differs in terms of cost, yield, accuracy, and practicality. Simple polymer blending and free radical copolymerization offer low-cost means to introduce functional chemical groups to surfaces and modify interfacial interactions. Biomolecules with diverse functionalities can be subsequently attached through linking reactions that occur either in the vapor phase or in solution. Encouragingly, most studies that report biomolecule immobilization on surfaces have observed successful attachment. Nevertheless, despite these promising short-term outcomes, very few studies have demonstrated long-term patency—an essential factor for the lasting success of implantable materials [70, 71].

8.4 Current Nanoengineered Constructs

A wide variety of nanoengineered structures have been developed so far, each representing a different phase of technological advancement. Nanotechnology has played a key role in enhancing their functionality, primarily by introducing nanoscale surface topographies that have significantly improved implant performance. These surface features can be engineered using specific chemical groups, nanoparticles, surface patterning, or a combination of these approaches. The following sections will outline and discuss notable examples of such engineered structures in greater detail.

8.4.1 Hollow Organs

In the development of artificial hollow organs like blood vessels and airways, nanoparticles, particularly polyhedral oligomeric silsesquioxane (POSS), have demonstrated enhanced performance in both in vitro and in vivo settings. For example, Seifalian et al. incorporated POSS into a proprietary polymer blend, achieving notable improvements in mechanical properties, including greater suture retention and enhanced thermal stability, even at a concentration as low as 2%. Atomic Force Microscopy (AFM) images show significant changes in surface texture, which promote cell adhesion and thus facilitate better implant integration. A nanocomposite trachea based on this material was successfully implanted in a patient under humanitarian grounds. The implant was found to be mechanically robust and effective in mucus clearance, while also supporting the regeneration of trachea-specific tissues. Similarly, blood vessels made from POSS-PCU have shown potential as alternatives to autologous grafts for both small and large-caliber vessels. The nanoengineered surface enhances endothelial cell attachment and growth, which has directed current research efforts toward developing drug-eluting models aimed at preventing the recurrence of atherosclerosis (Seifalian et al., unpublished data).

8.4.2 Bone and Cartilage

Orthopedic implants have perhaps seen the most significant advancements from nanoscale modifications (see Fig. 8.4). The enhanced adhesion of osteoblasts on nanostructured materials was first identified in 1999, with findings showing that titania with grain sizes between 32 and 56 nm and alumina ranging from 49 to 67 nm significantly outperformed their micro-grained versions in promoting osteoblast attachment. Subsequent investigations into nanoceramics, such as hydroxyapatite, titania, and alumina, revealed that when grain or fiber sizes were under 100 nm, these materials supported improved in vitro osteoblast proliferation and long-term functionality. This included elevated production of intracellular and extracellular matrix proteins like collagen and alkaline phosphatase, along with enhanced deposition of calcium-based minerals [72].

Additionally, nanofiber alumina structures showed even greater osteoblast performance, such as increased viable cell adhesion, proliferation, and calcium deposition, compared to nanospherical alumina. This improvement is believed to result from the nanofibers' structural resemblance to the collagen fibers and hydroxyapatite crystals naturally found in bone. Efforts in creating biomimetic polymer scaffolds for bone and cartilage repair have focused on incorporating hydroxyapatite into elastomeric

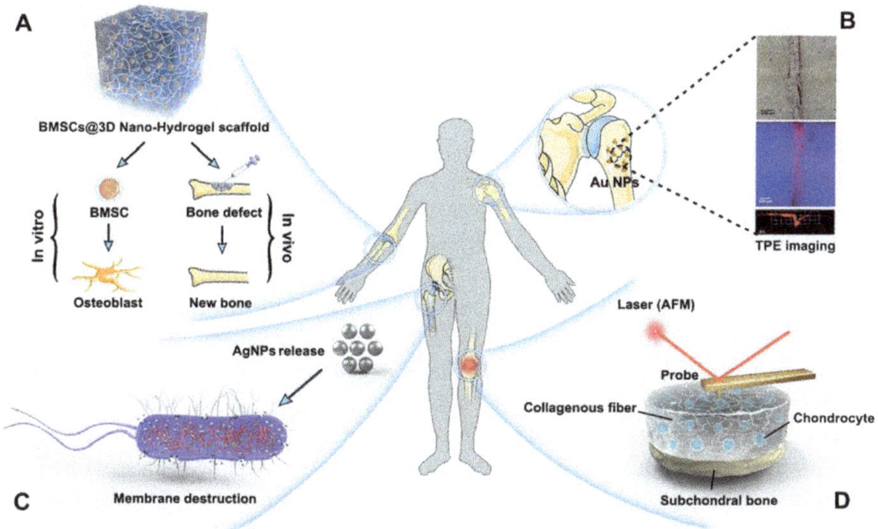

Fig. 8.4 Orthopedic applications of nanomedicine. **a** Development of innovative biomimetic nanomaterials for tissue repair. **b** Use of nanoparticle-based MRI contrast agents enables high-resolution, low-radiation imaging for diagnosing skeletal disorders. **c** Nanotechnology-driven design and synthesis of targeted drug delivery systems. **d** Utilization of atomic force microscopy (AFM) for early diagnosis and nanomechanical assessment of degenerative joint diseases. Figure reproduced under license CC BY 4.0 [73] (https://creativecommons.org/licenses/by/4.0/)

materials. Notable successes include the development of nasal and auricular scaffolds, considered the most promising results to date. 36 POSS-PCU scaffolds have been tested subcutaneously in rat models and, in a compassionate-use case, applied to a human arm. As mentioned earlier, the inclusion of POSS nanoparticles has led to improved cell attachment, proliferation, thermal stability, and suture retention, key factors for sterilization and successful implantation [74]. Research continues into further applications and scaffold development.

8.4.3 Dermal Grafts

Skin wounds remain a major healthcare and economic challenge. However, skin regeneration and replacement has been among the earliest and most successful applications of tissue engineering. Multiple FDA-approved skin substitutes are available for treating conditions like diabetic ulcers and severe burns. A well-known example is Apligraf® by Organogenesis, which is composed of a bilayer: human keratinocytes cultured atop a bovine collagen type I matrix and a layer of human dermal fibroblasts beneath [75]. While effective, such products are expensive mainly due to the prolonged in vitro culture time required for cell growth before they are ready for clinical use. Nanostructured scaffolds offer a promising alternative by reducing this culture period. For example, Chung et al. [76] developed a nanostructured chitosan (CS) film grafted onto poly(ε-caprolactone) (PCL), resulting in a surface roughness of 106 nm—significantly higher than the 3.6 nm of smooth CS/PCL. These nanostructures significantly enhanced fibroblast proliferation and viability, suggesting that solvent spin etching could be a cost-effective way to manufacture nanoengineered dermal grafts. In another approach, researchers in Singapore proposed **autologous layered dermal reconstitution (ALDR)** using electrospun PCL/gelatin fiber meshes (300–600 nm in diameter, 28 μm thick) [77]. Seeded with human dermal fibroblasts, the scaffolds supported cell proliferation over 14 days. While in vivo data is lacking, this method shows promise for rapid, layer-by-layer wound healing. Since electrospinning can be done directly on polyurethane wound dressings, it simplifies fabrication. However, electrospun meshes tend to have weaker mechanical properties. Dressings can be removed after 48–72 h and replaced, continuing until full wound closure. This approach eliminates the need for extended culture by seeding each scaffold with fibroblasts prior to application, enabling cellular infiltration and tissue growth across layers. Sun et al. [78] demonstrated that electrospun polystyrene scaffolds supported co-cultures of keratinocytes, fibroblasts, and endothelial cells, which organized into layers mimicking skin architecture. Co-culture extended viability beyond three days, unlike single-cell-type cultures. The nanoscale porosity was key, supporting faster vascularization compared to decellularized dermis, which lacks suitable pore structures. Finally, the Seifalian lab engineered multilayer nanocomposite dermal scaffolds, using a bottom-up strategy [79]. These contain POSS-enhanced PCL laminated with porous elastomer layers tailored to mimic native skin's varied topography and support multiple cell types. The prototype is currently undergoing in vivo testing against commercial products like Karoskin and Apligraf.

8.5 Current Position and 5-Year Outlook for Nano-enhanced Artificial Organs

The global tissue engineering market was valued at approximately USD 19.36 billion in 2024 and is expected to grow at a compound annual growth rate (CAGR) of 14.3% between 2025 and 2030 [80]. The rising incidence of chronic conditions such as cardiovascular diseases, diabetes, and orthopedic disorders has driven the demand for advanced tissue engineering approaches capable of repairing or replacing damaged tissues. Progress in areas such as biomaterials, 3D bioprinting, stem cell technology, and gene editing has significantly advanced the field. These innovations have enabled the development of complex, functional tissues, thereby increasing the likelihood of successful therapeutic applications.

Once considered a subset of biomaterials, tissue engineering has evolved into its own distinct industry, offering therapies that combine cells with engineered biochemical and physicochemical components to repair, enhance, or replace impaired biological functions. Over the past 30 years, interest in tissue engineering and cell therapies has steadily increased. While many specialized products remain in the research and development phase, some, such as wound dressings, have successfully transitioned from laboratory research to clinical use. Recently, large pharmaceutical and medical device companies have invested in smaller biotech firms, aiming to bring some of these therapies and devices to commercial viability. Additionally, many smaller companies have been acquired by larger corporations looking to integrate these technologies into their portfolios. Despite millions of dollars in private funding directed annually toward research and development, it often takes over a decade to advance a product to human clinical trials. Due to the high financial demands of development, many smaller companies have been forced to close or sell their promising innovations and intellectual property to larger organizations.

8.6 Developmental Timescales

Developing tissue engineering and cellular therapy products requires years of research and substantial financial investment, averaging around $300 million annually in recent times, before they can successfully pass regulatory approvals, undergo clinical trials, and become available for medical use. Small biotech companies often quickly exhaust their funds and struggle to secure sufficient financing to continue operations. Although large pharmaceutical and medical device companies actively monitor progress and frequently collaborate or enter licensing agreements with leading biotech firms, they remain cautious about funding product development due to the high risks involved, as many products may never achieve commercial success. Most of the products currently in development are expected to be launched within the next ten to twenty years, with the exception of some skin, bone, and cartilage products already on the market. Since European regulatory approval processes are generally less stringent than those of the FDA, many products may debut in Europe before reaching the US. However, launching a product does not guarantee widespread patient adoption, as tissue engineering and cell therapy products will initially be reserved for patients with severe conditions like cancer or those urgently needing organ transplants. Treatment decisions will also be influenced by insurance coverage, cautious family members, and conservative physicians' hesitancy. More progressive doctors, informed by firsthand experience, patient outcomes, and peer discussions, will carefully select patients for these therapies. In essence, the adoption of tissue engineering and cellular therapies will follow the typical pattern for new technologies: cautious and specialized use by knowledgeable physicians dedicated to providing optimal patient care without undue risk. Consequently, it will take additional time for these products to become well-established and routinely used in clinical practice.

8.7 Conclusions and Future Directions

With numerous products currently in clinical trials and late-stage development, promising results, and ongoing financial investment, nanotechnology is poised to significantly influence the future of medicine. However, the transition from laboratory research to clinical application is far from straightforward. While nanotechnology is driving progress in artificial organ development, many challenges and safety concerns remain to be addressed. Moreover, a comprehensive evaluation of the potential for chemical surface modifications is essential. Since surface chemistry alterations are both versatile and cost-effective, they could represent the final hurdle in achieving the ideal artificial organ.

References

1. Ellahi A, Gupta S, Bose D, Chanda A (2025) A high-fidelity biomechanical modeling framework for injury prediction during frontal car crash. Comput Methods Biomech Biomed Eng 28:13–24
2. Gupta S, Singh G, Chanda A (2021) Prediction of diabetic foot ulcer progression: a computational study. Biomed Phys Eng Express 7:065020
3. Gupta S, Gupta V, Chanda A (2022) Biomechanical modeling of novel high expansion auxetic skin grafts. Int J Numer Method Biomed Eng 38:e3586
4. Anjum S et al (2021) Emerging applications of nanotechnology in healthcare systems: grand challenges and perspectives. Pharmaceuticals (Basel) 14:707
5. Jaiswal JK, Simon SM (2004) Potentials and pitfalls of fluorescent quantum dots for biological imaging. Trends Cell Biol 14:497–504
6. Chanda A, Gupta S (2025) Healthcare entrepreneurship and management. Routledge, Taylor & Francis Group
7. Afazal M, Gupta S, Tevatia A, Afreen S, Chanda A (2023) Computational fluid dynamics-based model for assessing rupture risk in cerebral arteries with varying aneurysm sizes. Computation 11:79
8. Ballou B et al (2007) Sentinel lymph node imaging using quantum dots in mouse tumor models. Bioconjug Chem 18:389–396
9. Yadav P, Kamboj M, Das B (2024) Application of nanotechnology in antimicrobial coating on surgical instruments. In: Applications of nanotechnology in biomedical engineering, pp 150–168. https://doi.org/10.1201/9781003432661-9
10. Voura EB, Jaiswal JK, Mattoussi H, Simon SM (2004) Tracking metastatic tumor cell extravasation with quantum dot nanocrystals and fluorescence emission-scanning microscopy. Nat Med 10:993–998
11. Yadav P et al (2025) Gelatin multiwalled carbon nanotube composite 3D printed semi biological mesh for abdominal hernia treatment. Chem Asian J 20:e202401136
12. Schroeder JE, Shweky I, Shmeeda H, Banin U, Gabizon A (2007) Folate-mediated tumor cell uptake of quantum dots entrapped in lipid nanoparticles. J Control Release 124:28–34
13. Yoshioka T et al (2011) Fate of bone marrow mesenchymal stem cells following the allogeneic transplantation of cartilaginous aggregates into osteochondral defects of rabbits. J Tissue Eng Regen Med 5:437–443
14. Singh G, Yadav P, Chanda A (2024) Development of biofidelic skin simulants based on fresh cadaveric skin tests. Eur Burn J 5:454–463
15. Verma S, Domb AJ, Kumar N (2011) Nanomaterials for regenerative medicine. Nanomedicine (London) 6:157–181

16. Verma S, Singh G, Chanda A (2023) A novel finite element model for the study of harmful vibrations on the aging spine. Computation 11:93
17. Hervault A, Thanh NTK (2014) Magnetic nanoparticle-based therapeutic agents for thermo-chemotherapy treatment of cancer. Nanoscale 6:11553–11573
18. Pacak CA et al (2014) Superparamagnetic iron oxide nanoparticles function as a long-term, multi-modal imaging label for non-invasive tracking of implanted progenitor cells. PLoS ONE 9
19. Verma S, Singh G, Chanda A (2024) Development of a computational framework for determination of detrimental vibrations on the human spine segments. Multiscale Sci Eng 6(4):48–56
20. Verma S, Chanda A (2024) State-of-the-art of finite element modelling of the human spine to study the impact of vibrations: a review. Int J Comput Methods Eng Sci Mech 25:225–247
21. Cheng K et al (2014) Magnetic antibody-linked nanomatchmakers for therapeutic cell targeting. Nat Commun 5:1–9
22. Kannan RY, Salacinski HJ, Odlyha M, Butler PE, Seifalian AM (2006) The degradative resistance of polyhedral oligomeric silsesquioxane nanocore integrated polyurethanes: an in vitro study. Biomaterials 27:1971–1979
23. Singh G, Chanda A (2022) Biomechanical modeling of progressive wound healing: a computational study. Biomed Eng Adv 4:100055
24. Gupta V, Chanda A (2024) Mechanical characterization of alternating slit, I-shaped and rotating triangle based auxetic skin graft phantoms. Mech Adv Mater Struct. https://doi.org/10.1080/15376494.2023.2250782
25. Bose D, Gupta S, Chanda A (2025) Scalable direct manufacturing of a functional multipurpose wrist-hand orthosis using 3D printing. Ann 3D Print Med 17:100186
26. Gu X, Wu J, Mather PT (2011) Polyhedral oligomeric silsesquioxane (POSS) suppresses enzymatic degradation of PCL-based polyurethanes. Biomacromol 12:3066–3077
27. Chanda A, Gupta V, Gupta S (2024) Development and mechanical testing of auxetic incisions on human cadaveric skin, pp 89–99. https://doi.org/10.1007/978-981-97-4383-4_7
28. Singh G, Gupta V, Chanda A (2022) Artificial skin with varying biomechanical properties. Mater Today Proc 62:3162–3166
29. Gupta V, Chanda A (2023) Auxetic incisions with alternating slit shapes: a promising technique for enhancing synthetic skin grafts expansion. Mater Res Express 10:075802
30. Chanda A, Upchurch W (2018) Biomechanical modeling of wounded skin. J Compos Sci 2:69
31. Loman-Cortes P, Huq TB, Vivero-Escoto JL (2021) Use of polyhedral oligomeric silsesquioxane (POSS) in drug delivery, photodynamic therapy and bioimaging. Molecules 26:6453
32. Shameli K, Bin Ahmad M, Zargar M, Yunus WMZW, Ibrahim NA (2011) Fabrication of silver nanoparticles doped in the zeolite framework and antibacterial activity. Int J Nanomed 6:331
33. Xin L, Wang J, Wu Y, Guo S, Tong J (2015) Increased oxidative stress and activated heat shock proteins in human cell lines by silver nanoparticles. Hum Exp Toxicol 34:315–323
34. Holbrook RD, Rykaczewski K, Staymates ME (2014) Dynamics of silver nanoparticle release from wound dressings revealed via in situ nanoscale imaging. J Mater Sci Mater Med 25:2481–2489
35. Gupta V, Singla R, Chanda A (2023) Development and characterization of novel anisotropic skin graft simulants. Dermato 3:114–130
36. Jiang C et al (2022) Biomechanics of skin grafts: effect of pattern size, spacing and orientation. Eng Res Express 4:015006
37. Gupta V, Singh G, Chanda A (2023) Modeling of metamaterial based incision patterns for generating high expansions in skin grafts. Clin Biomech 110:106118
38. Singh G, Chanda A (2024) Development and biomechanical testing of artificial surrogates for vaginal tissue. Adv Mater Process Technol. https://doi.org/10.1080/2374068X.2023.2198837
39. Iijima S (1991) Helical microtubules of graphitic carbon. Nature 354:56–58
40. Iijima S, Ichihashi T (1993) Single-shell carbon nanotubes of 1-nm diameter. Nature 363:603–605

41. Baughman RH et al (1999) Carbon nanotube actuators. Science (80-) 284:1340–1344
42. Nezakati T, Cousins BG, Seifalian AM (2014) Toxicology of chemically modified graphene-based materials for medical application. Arch Toxicol 88:1987–2012
43. Gupta V, Singh G, Chanda A, Chanda A (2021) Expansion potential of skin grafts with novel I-shaped auxetic incisions. Biomed Phys Eng Express 8:015016
44. Chanda A, Chatterjee S, Gupta V (2020) Soft composite based hyperelastic model for anisotropic tissue characterization. J Compos Mater 54:4525–4534
45. Singh G, Gupta V, Chanda A (2022) Mechanical characterization of rotating triangle shaped auxetic skin graft simulants. Facta Univ Ser Mech Eng
46. Nezakati T, Tan A, Seifalian AM (2014) Enhancing the electrical conductivity of a hybrid POSS–PCL/graphene nanocomposite polymer. J Colloid Interface Sci 435:145–155
47. Chhikara K, Gupta S, Chanda A (2022) Development of a novel foot orthosis for plantar pain reduction. Mater Today Proc 62:3532–3537
48. Chanda A, Unnikrishnan V, Flynn Z, Lackey K (2017) Experimental study on tissue phantoms to understand the effect of injury and suturing on human skin mechanical properties. Proc Inst Mech Eng Part H J Eng Med 231:80–91
49. Chanda A (2018) Biomechanical modeling of human skin tissue surrogates. Biomimetics 3
50. Chhikara K, Sidhu SS, Gupta S, Saharawat S, Kataria C, Chanda A (2023) Development and effectiveness testing of a novel 3D-printed multi-material orthosis in nurses with plantar foot pain. Prosthesis 5:73–87
51. Accioni F, Vázquez J, Merinero M, Begines B, Alcudia A (2022) Latest trends in surface modification for dental implantology: innovative developments and analytical applications. Pharmaceutics 14(2):455
52. Newman KD, Elamanchili P, Kwon GS, Samuel J (2002) Protein and surface effects on monocyte and macrophage adhesion, maturation, and survival. J Biomed Mater Res 60:487–496
53. Fisher JP, Mikos AG, Bronzino JD (1993) Tissue engineering. Science 260:1–583
54. Gupta V, Singh G, Gupta S, Chanda A (2023) Expansion potential of auxetic prosthetic skin grafts: a review. Eng. Res. Express 5:022003
55. Gupta V, Chanda A (2023) Biomechanical modelling of hierarchical metamaterials for skin grafting. Mater Horizons Nat Nanomater Part F 1471:71–83
56. Chanda A, Flynn Z, Unnikrishnan V (2018) Biomechanical characterization of normal and prolapsed vaginal tissue surrogates. J Mech Med Biol 18(6):1750100. https://doi.org/10.1142/S0219519417501007
57. Afazal M, Afreen S, Chanda A (2023) Computational modelling and analysis of hard tissue behavior around 0.5 mm and 0.85 mm platform switched abutment using 3D finite element analysis. Forces Mech13:100243
58. Wang Y, Kim HJ, Vunjak-Novakovic G, Kaplan DL (2006) Stem cell-based tissue engineering with silk biomaterials. Biomaterials 27:6064–6082
59. Devine C, McCollum C (2004) Heparin-bonded Dacron or polytetrafluorethylene for femoropopliteal bypass: five-year results of a prospective randomized multicenter clinical trial. J Vasc Surg 40:924–931
60. Chanda A, Ruchti T, Unnikrishnan V (2018) Computational modeling of wound suture: a review. IEEE Rev Biomed Eng 11:165–176
61. Gupta V, Singh G, Chanda A (2023) Development of hierarchical auxetic skin graft simulants with high expansion potential. Biomed Eng Adv 5:100087
62. Rothschild BM et al (2023) Design, manufacturing, and trial of a 3D printed customized finger splint for patients with rheumatoid arthritis. Rheumato 3:51–62
63. Singh G, Chanda A (2024) Finite element modeling of diabetic foot: a state-of-the-art review. Eng Res Express 6:012507
64. Hergenrother RW, Cooper SL (1992) Improved materials for blood-contacting applications: blends of sulphonated and non-sulphonated polyurethanes. J Mater Sci Mater Med 3:313–321
65. Recek N et al (2013) Protein adsorption on various plasma-treated polyethylene terephthalate substrates. Molecules 18:12441

66. Alves P et al (2014) Improving cell adhesion: development of a biosensor for cell behaviour monitoring by surface grafting of sulfonic groups onto a thermoplastic polyurethane. J Mater Sci Mater Med 25:2017–2026
67. Xiao S et al (2021) Bi-layer silk fibroin skeleton and bladder acellular matrix hydrogel encapsulating adipose-derived stem cells for bladder reconstruction. Biomater Sci 9:6169–6182
68. Plasma Phys 670 (2005)
69. Hoshi RA et al (2013) The blood and vascular cell compatibility of heparin-modified ePTFE vascular grafts. Biomaterials 34:30–41
70. Singh G, Chanda A (2024) Biofidelic gallbladder tissue surrogates. Adv Mater Process Technol. https://doi.org/10.1080/2374068X.2023.2198835
71. Majumdar P, Singh G, Chanda A (2024) Development and biomechanical testing of full-scale human brain simulant. J Eng Res. https://doi.org/10.1016/J.JER.2024.02.016
72. Webster TJ, Siegel RW, Bizios R (1999) Osteoblast adhesion on nanophase ceramics. Biomaterials 20:1221–1227
73. Qiao K et al (2022) The advances in nanomedicine for bone and cartilage repair. J Nanobiotechnol 20:1–42
74. Webster TJ, Ergun C, Doremus RH, Siegel RW, Bizios R (2000) Enhanced functions of osteoblasts on nanophase ceramics. Biomaterials 21:1803–1810
75. Eaglstein WH, Falanga V (1997) Tissue engineering and the development of Apligraf®, a human skin equivalent. Clin Ther 19:894–905
76. Chung TW, Wang YZ, Huang YY, Pan CI, Wang SS (2006) Poly(ε-caprolactone) grafted with nano-structured chitosan enhances growth of human dermal fibroblasts. Artif Organs 30:35–41
77. Chong EJ et al (2007) Evaluation of electrospun PCL/gelatin nanofibrous scaffold for wound healing and layered dermal reconstitution. Acta Biomater 3:321–330
78. Sun T et al (2005) Self-organization of skin cells in three-dimensional electrospun polystyrene scaffolds. Tissue Eng 11:1023–1033
79. Chawla R et al (2014) A polyhedral oligomeric silsesquioxane-based bilayered dermal scaffold seeded with adipose tissue-derived stem cells: In vitro assessment of biomechanical properties. J Surg Res 188:361–372
80. Tissue engineering market size and share report, 2030. https://www.grandviewresearch.com/industry-analysis/tissue-engineering-and-regeneration-industry

Chapter 9
3D-Printed Artificial Tissues

The invention of the printing press in the fifteenth century revolutionized information dissemination by enabling rapid, cost-effective reproduction of text, fostering innovation and access to knowledge [1]. Bioprinting, similarly transformative, offers a high-throughput, affordable method for assembling complex tissues by using additive manufacturing techniques to pattern cells, biomaterials, and biomolecules [2–4]. This technology leverages bio-inks, the biocompatible materials that act as scaffolds to support printed cells, which are then matured in bioreactors. Bioprinting holds significant potential for advancing tissue engineering and regenerative medicine by creating custom tissue constructs for transplantation and research [5]. It enables the precise fabrication of 3D structures that mimic the complexity of natural tissues, facilitating breakthroughs in developmental biology, drug testing, and precision medicine. By replicating the extracellular and cellular components of tissues, bioprinting can address the growing need for model systems and personalized medical applications [6]. As bioprinting evolves, integrating advances in fundamental sciences, materials science, and robotics will drive innovative solutions to current challenges in regenerative medicine. The development of bio-inspired materials and improved bioprinting platforms will enhance the ability to replicate tissue functions and structures. Future research aims to expand the scope of biological applications, ultimately transforming the field of tissue engineering [7, 8]. This chapter highlights recent advances in bioprinting, focusing on its methodologies, applications, and future directions, emphasizing its potential to reshape regenerative medicine and tissue engineering.

A. Chanda and D. Sharma, *Handbook of Artificial Tissues, Biofabrication and Bioprinting, Volume I*, Biomedical Materials for Multi-functional Applications,
https://doi.org/10.1007/978-981-92-1307-8_9

9.1 Bioprinting Industry

The growing economic potential of 3D bioprinting is driving its rapid shift from academic research to a burgeoning industry. This technology shows promise across multiple sectors, including tissue transplantation, precision medicine, and drug development. By 2021, the 3D printing market, valued at \$2.2 billion in 2012, was expected to reach \$10.8 billion [9]. As of 2014, around 30 companies worldwide were actively involved in 3D bioprinting, focusing on bioprinters and bioprinted scaffolds for research and commercial purposes. Currently, there are more than seven types of 3D bioprinters tailored for academic and industrial R&D. These devices primarily rely on two techniques: droplet-based and extrusion-based bioprinting. Companies like Tissue Regeneration Systems have pioneered patient-specific bone regeneration solutions using bioprinted polycaprolactone (PCL) scaffolds, earning FDA approval in 2013 for the first 3D bioprinted implant in skeletal repair. Similarly, a bioprinted liver tissue was designed for drug toxicity testing. Despite its utility in preclinical drug screening, significant challenges remain in developing fully functional and commercially viable liver tissues [10–13]. Several bioprinting companies also offer specialized software, such as TSIM®, BioAssemblyBot®, and BioCAD®, to support the design and fabrication of complex tissue structures. These tools enhance the precision and scalability of bioprinting, facilitating the creation of multiscale biological models from individual cells to entire tissues. Overall, the field continues to grow, driven by innovations in both hardware and software, with the potential to transform biomedical applications [14–16].

9.2 Advanced Bioprinting Materials and Technology

Three primary methods are employed for 3D printing biological materials, including cells, growth factors, and hydrogels: droplet-based bioprinting, laser-based bioprinting, and extrusion-based bioprinting [17–19]. Each technique has distinct features influencing outcomes, such as cell viability and functionality after printing. The mechanics and parameters of bioprinting methods are covered in further detail in this section.

9.2.1 Droplet Bioprinting

Droplet bioprinting, one of the earliest methods used in tissue and organ fabrication, operates by depositing cell-laden droplets layer by layer onto a substrate using a non-contact technique [20]. Droplet generation relies on either piezoelectric or thermal mechanisms [21]. In thermal droplet bioprinting, heat is applied to the bio-ink chamber, creating pressure pulses that eject picoliter-sized droplets through the nozzle. In contrast, piezoelectric bioprinters use acoustic waves generated by a piezoelectric crystal actuator to expel droplets. This method offers several advantages, including low cost, high precision at the microscale, rapid printing speeds (up to 10 kHz), and good post-printing cell viability [22]. It is also compatible with hydrogels and other nonliving materials, contributing to its widespread adoption. Figure 9.1 shows the reactive jet impingement system consisting of an in-house developed printhead integrated with a JetLab 4 XL (MicroFab Technologies, USA) printing workstation [23]. However, there are several limitations, such as printing high-viscosity materials or bio-inks with dense cell concentrations, which can lead to nozzle clogging, posing challenges for tissue fabrication. Additionally, using low-viscosity bio-inks can compromise the mechanical integrity of printed structures, complicating the creation of fully functional 3D tissues. Despite these challenges, droplet bioprinting remains a promising tool for applications requiring precision and speed in tissue engineering [24].

9.2.2 Laser Bioprinting

Laser bioprinting, which utilizes the laser-induced forward transfer (LIFT) technique, is an advanced method for fabricating tissues and positioning living cells [25]. Figure 9.2 shows the schematic representation of the experimental setup for LIFT of cell spheroids [26]. In this process, a pulsed laser beam is directed at a specialized ribbon, a glass slide coated with a polyimide membrane, titanium, or gold layer that absorbs the laser's energy. The ribbon holds the bio-ink, which contains cells and biological materials [27]. As a nozzle-free technique, laser bioprinting can handle bio-inks with high viscosities and cell densities, avoiding issues like clogging and excessive heat buildup common in droplet and extrusion-based methods. Despite these advantages, several challenges have limited its broader application. The high cost of laser bioprinters and the narrow beam width, which restricts the ability to print large structures, are significant barriers. Additionally, the method's low flow rate is a limitation, as rapid gelation is required to maintain high-resolution and precise structures [28]. Another drawback is the potential for metallic residues from the evaporated laser-absorbing layer to contaminate the final tissue constructs. These challenges highlight the need for further innovation to make laser bioprinting more scalable and cost-effective for tissue engineering applications.

9.2.3 Extrusion Bioprinting

Extrusion bioprinting is one of the most widely used and cost-effective methods for tissue biofabrication. The system consists of a dispensing mechanism, either mechanical (piston or screw-based) or pneumatic, and a robotic platform with three-axis (x–y–z) control, managed by a stage controller [29–32]. This technique works by

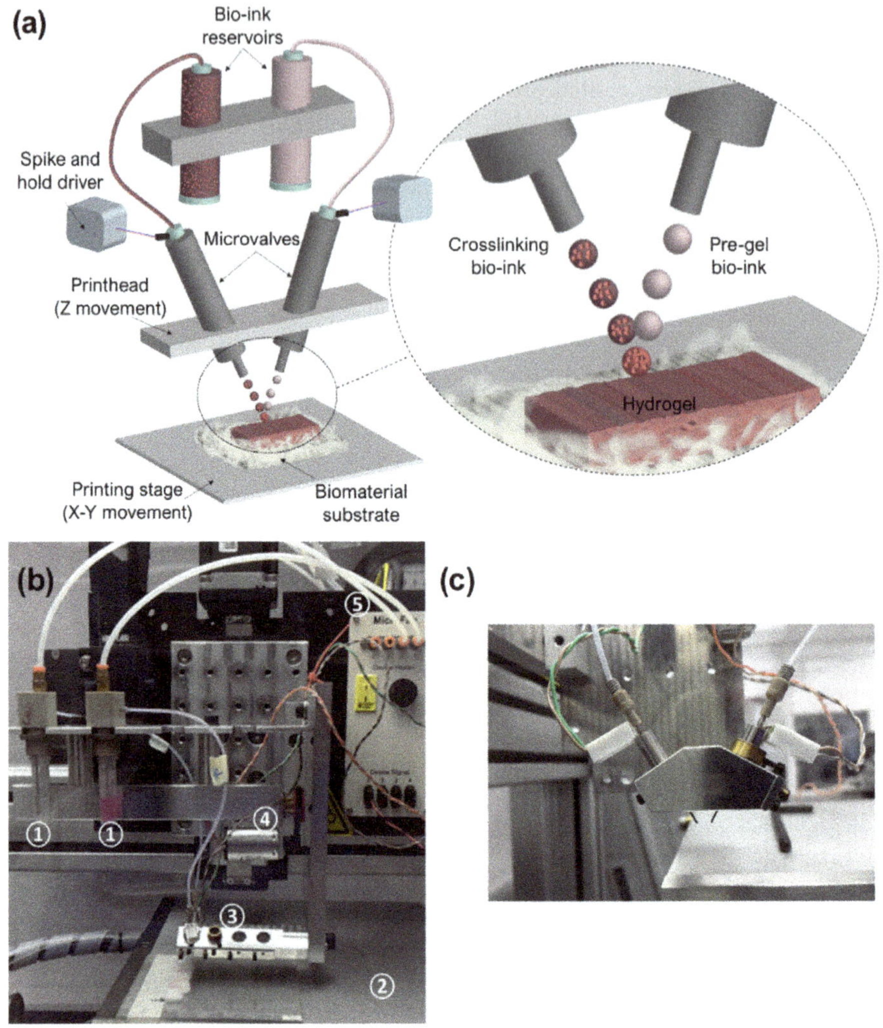

Fig. 9.1 **a** Schematic representation of reactive jet impingement setup (ReJI); **b** components of ReJI setup: (1) bio-ink reservoirs; (2) printer stage; (3) printhead with valves; (4) motor system responsible for cell agitation; (5) pressure tubing system; **c** ReJI printhead with a pair of microvalves. Figure reproduced under license CC-BY-4.0 [23] (https://creativecommons.org/licenses/by/4.0/)

depositing bio-ink containing suspended cells onto a substrate in a continuous stream rather than discrete droplets. A key advantage of extrusion bioprinting is its ability to print bio-inks with high viscosities and cell densities at relatively high speeds while maintaining good cell viability [33]. Figure 9.3 showcases sample images of various alginate-gelatin ink formulations being manually dispensed alongside the corresponding scaffolds printed using these inks. In particular, the 4% and 6% alginate concentrations formed droplets instead of continuous fibers when dispensed

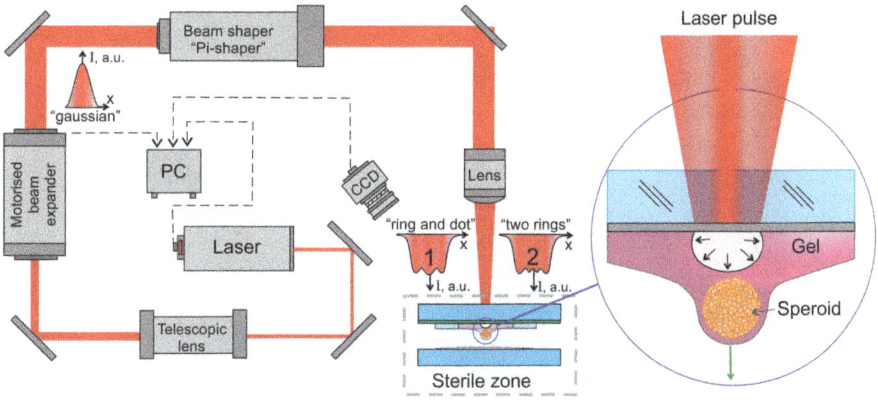

Fig. 9.2 Experimental setup for laser bioprinting with cell spheroids. On the right, a cell spheroid shows the start of its transfer using a bio-ink jet. Figure reproduced under license CC-BY-4.0 [26] (https://creativecommons.org/licenses/by/4.0/)

through the syringe's bioprinting nozzle. Structural images of the resulting scaffolds further validate the printability and suitability of these inks for scaffold fabrication [34, 35]. However, it has limitations in resolution, achieving only around 200 μm. Mechanical dispensers offer precise control over material flow but can expose cells to shear stress, potentially causing deformation. In contrast, pneumatic dispensers reduce cell damage but face challenges in maintaining accurate material flow due to delays in compressed gas regulation [36–38]. To address these issues, nozzle-free acoustic bioprinting has been developed, enabling precise cell encapsulation at picoliter scales while avoiding nozzle clogging. This advancement enhances cell viability and accuracy. Extrusion bioprinting also opens up new applications, such as preserving cells for transfusion medicine and studying single cells for regenerative medicine and omics research [39].

9.3 Bioprinting Materials/Bio-Inks

Replicating the architecture and composition of native tissues using 3D bioprinting is challenging, as it requires a thorough understanding of cell physiology and interactions with the extracellular matrix (ECM). Achieving a balance between the physical and chemical signals influencing cells involves selecting appropriate biomaterials. These can include natural materials such as collagen, fibrin, hydroxyapatite, and hyaluronic acid (HA), as well as synthetic options like polycaprolactone (PCL), polylactide (PLA), polyglycolide (PGA), poly(lactic-co-glycolic acid) (PLGA), and polyethylene glycol (PEG). Hybrid biomaterials, which combine natural and synthetic components, can also be used to engineer 3D microenvironments tailored to support specific cellular functions [40–43].

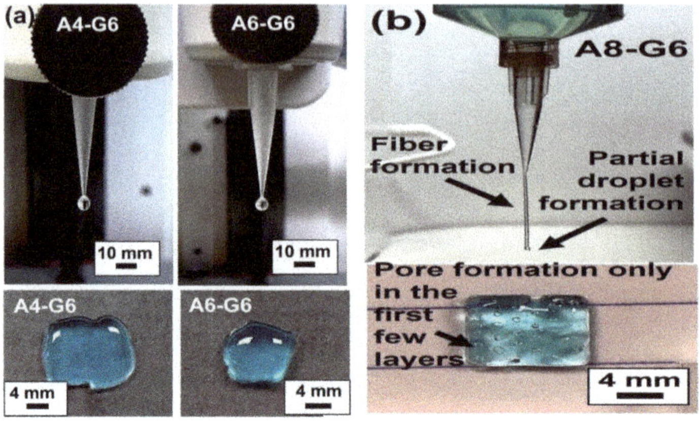

Fig. 9.3 Inks and the corresponding scaffolds: **a** A4-G6 and A6-G6 ink droplets when extruded out of the nozzle. No structural and shape fidelity was observed with these printed scaffolds; **b** A8-G6 inks formed partial fiber formation and droplets with satisfactory shape and structural fidelity. Figure reproduced under license CC-BY-4.0 [34] (https://creativecommons.org/licenses/by/4.0/)

9.3.1 Natural Materials

The chemical and physical properties of natural hydrogels can be tailored based on the target tissue and cell types, as factors like stiffness, viscosity, and porosity are crucial for the survival and functionality of bioprinted constructs. Many cell types can degrade natural hydrogels and produce their own extracellular matrix (ECM), allowing for cell migration and proliferation [44]. These hydrogels can also be engineered to include tissue-specific growth factors and chemokines, such as matrix metalloproteinases, insulin-like growth factor, epidermal growth factor, and transforming growth factor beta (TGF-β), to restore the microenvironment's chemical signals [45]. However, batch-to-batch variability in natural hydrogels can affect consistency and compromise the validation of the designed microenvironment. Collagen and fibrinogen-based hydrogels are widely used in tissue engineering, with collagen type I being the most common ECM component, promoting cell adhesion and 3D growth. Gelatin methacrylate (GelMA), a photocrosslinkable hydrogel, supports proteolytic degradation and integrin-mediated cell attachment, making it a versatile option for artificial tissue creation due to its ease of manipulation and crosslinking. Alginate, a biocompatible polymer, is often used in 3D bioprinting due to its ability to crosslink in calcium solutions. Additionally, reconstituted basement membranes, such as Matrigel™ and Cultrex®, derived from mouse tumors, contain key ECM proteins like collagen IV, fibronectin, and laminin [46]. These membranes enhance cell adhesion and spatial organization, supporting 3D cell cultures and improving cell activity when incorporated into bioprinting polymer solutions [47].

9.3.2 *Synthetic and Semi-synthetic Materials*

To address the limitations of biologically derived biomaterials, such as batch-to-batch variability, a range of synthetic and semi-synthetic biomaterials has been developed. These materials, engineered to include natural ECM components and customizable properties, enhance reproducibility and comparability across experiments, making them suitable for bioprinting applications. Commonly used biocompatible synthetic polymers in tissue engineering include polycaprolactone (PCL), polyethylene glycol (PEG), polylactide (PLA), polyglycolide (PGA), and poly(lactic-co-glycolic acid) (PLGA) [48]. PEG hydrogels are among the most widely utilized synthetic matrices. These hydrogels can be chemically or UV-crosslinked using functionalized polymers, enabling effective cell encapsulation. PEG-based hydrogels can also be biomimetic by incorporating bioactive ligands, such as oligopeptides or full protein growth factors, to restore biochemical signaling. For example, including arginine–glycine–aspartic acid (RGD) peptides promotes integrin-mediated cell attachment and motility [49]. However, synthetic matrices lack the native ECM's complex biochemical cues, making them less physiologically relevant than naturally derived 3D matrices. Self-assembled peptide hydrogels are another innovation, creating 3D cell culture environments through peptide sequences that form stable scaffolds [50–52]. These scaffolds offer sufficient mechanical strength, making them suitable for tissue engineering, particularly in bone tissue culture. PCL stands out as a promising bio-ink for orthopedic applications due to its mechanical stability. The osteogenic properties of PCL-based constructs can be enhanced by incorporating osteoinductive hydroxyapatite particles, improving stiffness and promoting bone-like characteristics [53]. Complex 3D structures can also be fabricated by layering cell-loaded alginate onto hydroxyapatite-based bio-inks. The resulting scaffolds combine mechanical strength and biological functionality, making them ideal for bone tissue engineering. Overall, synthetic and semi-synthetic biomaterials, such as PEG hydrogels, self-assembled peptide scaffolds, and PCL composites, offer significant potential for enhancing the mechanical and biological performance of 3D bioprinted scaffolds. Their customizable properties and compatibility with bioprinting technologies pave the way for innovative biomedical applications, especially in regenerative medicine and tissue engineering [54–56].

9.4 Biomedical Applications

9.4.1 *Bioprinting for Tissue Regeneration and Regenerative Medicine*

Various bioprinting techniques have shown the potential of additive manufacturing to create tissue models that could be used for tissue fabrication. This includes successfully printing several organs and tissues, such as the heart, liver, kidneys, skin, neurons, and vascular networks. Key approaches for constructing 3D-printed tissue structures while maintaining their biological functions are outlined in this section [38, 57–66].

9.4.2 *Vascular Grafts*

The challenge of vascularization, which impacts mass transfer, oxygen diffusion, and nutrient delivery in vivo, remains a significant barrier in tissue engineering. Vascular grafts have become a key focus in 3D bioprinting research due to their crucial role in addressing this issue. These grafts were developed using a "scaffold-free" bioprinting approach [66], where cell spheroids and agarose templates were utilized to construct tubular structures. Multicellular spheroids, formed using agarose molds, were assembled into tubular shapes, acting as structural building blocks. In Fig. 9.4, the cell-laden alginate bio-ink was crosslinked by lowering the stage and submerging the structure in a $CaCl_2$ solution [67]. To enhance its long-term stability, the printed structure underwent additional crosslinking with barium chloride. Human aortic smooth muscle cells, aortic endothelial cells, and dermal fibroblasts were also employed to fabricate vascular grafts. During the post-printing phase, the cells were allowed to fuse, as depicted. The grafts were then placed in a bioreactor to undergo a maturation process to improve their mechanical and physical properties. In another approach, vascular channels were created using 3D bioprinting combined with perfusion techniques [68–70]. Human umbilical vein endothelial cells (HUVECs) were printed using a collagen hydrogel precursor, with gelatin used to form the vascular grafts. These printed structures were incorporated into a polycarbonate flow chamber to generate functional fluidic grafts. Viability tests confirmed that these grafts demonstrated enhanced cell viability under dynamic flow conditions.

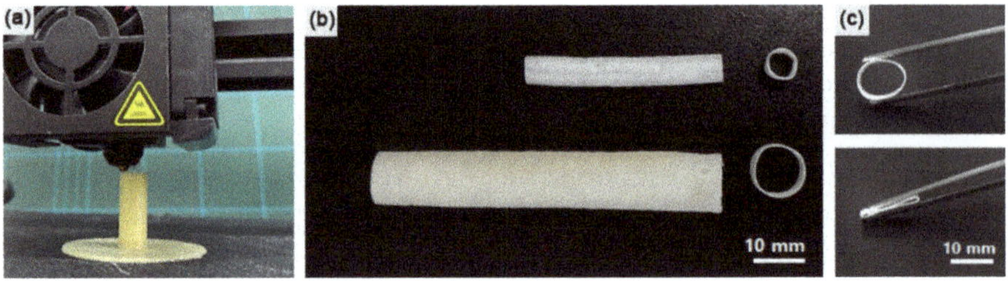

Fig. 9.4 3D printed vascular graft model. Figure reproduced under license CC-BY-4.0 [67] (https://creativecommons.org/licenses/by/4.0/)

9.4.3 Skin

Skin tissue bioprinting holds significant promise for applications such as topical drug development, wound healing studies, and cutaneous toxicity assessments. Various approaches have been explored to replicate the physiology and cellular microenvironment of human skin. For instance, laser-assisted bioprinting has been used to deposit fibroblasts and keratinocytes onto a stabilizing matrix (Matriderm) for the creation of skin substitutes. Both in vitro and in vivo trials suggest that this method can promote neovascularization. In another study, amniotic fluid-derived stem cells (AFSCs) were printed using a direct-forward bioprinting technique to support skin regeneration and wound healing in a mouse model. The process involved combining bone marrow-derived mesenchymal stem cells (MSCs) and AFSCs in a fibrin-collagen matrix [71]. By the second week, wounds treated with the MSC and AFSC mixture exhibited the formation of a distinct and well-organized epidermal layer, unlike those treated with gel alone, which showed poor epidermal development. Fluorescent labeling indicated that the printed cells remained localized and did not migrate into the surrounding regenerated tissue [72–76].

9.4.4 Neuron

3D bioprinting of neural cells is ideal for modeling neural diseases, regeneration, and complex networks, as well as for exploring new therapeutic strategies, including treatments for Parkinson's and Alzheimer's diseases. However, a significant challenge lies in replicating the brain's intricate, multilayered structure, particularly along the medial or sagittal plane. Additionally, creating functional neural tissues post-printing remains difficult. Recent advancements include using an extrusion-based 3D bioprinter to fabricate multilayered brain-like structures composed of primary brain cells embedded in a natural hydrogel derived from gellan gum modified with RGD peptides [77–79]. The resulting structure mimics cortical tissue. After five days in culture, confocal microscopy revealed the formation of 3D brain networks, with no significant difference in cell viability between printed and control groups over the same period [80, 81]. In another study, a piezoelectric droplet bioprinter was used to pattern retinal ganglion cell (RGC) neurons and retinal glial cells from adult rats. Neurite outgrowth and cell viability were comparable between printed and control cells. Notably, RGC neurons exhibited enhanced expansion when glial cells were used as a substrate [82]. A novel bioacoustic levitation assembly (BAL) technique was also developed to create 3D brain-like structures. Human neural progenitor cells (hNPCs) were suspended and positioned at acoustic standing wave nodes within a fibrinogen solution using acoustic radiation forces [83]. The interlayer spacing could be precisely controlled by adjusting the acoustic frequency, and the gelation process immobilized the cells within a fibrin hydrogel, allowing them to differentiate and form both intra- and inter-layer neural connections in the 3D environment.

This BAL method offers a fast, biocompatible way to engineer multilayered tissue constructs with potential applications in cancer research, cardiovascular studies, and neurology.

9.4.5 Bone

Bone regeneration research often encounters challenges related to graft porosity and vascularization. Gene therapy has emerged as a promising approach for delivering therapeutic agents to target sites and enhancing bone repair [84]. A novel technique has been developed that integrates gene therapy with advanced bioprinting methods. Specifically, plasmid DNA encoding bone morphogenetic protein-2 (BMP-2) is incorporated into the bioprinted constructs to promote osteogenic differentiation. Porous structures demonstrated superior BMP-2 production compared to non-porous ones, with porosity playing a crucial role in accelerating osteogenic differentiation. Both porous and BMP-2-enriched constructs exhibited increased levels of osteogenic markers, such as alkaline phosphatase and osteocalcin, creating an optimal environment for bone regeneration [85]. Another innovative approach utilizes a nanoliter gel droplet system combined with bioprinting to mimic a biomimetic fibrocartilage microenvironment. In this method, human mesenchymal stem cells (MSCs) are encapsulated in a gelatin-based methacrylated hydrogel bio-ink. BMP-2 and transforming growth factor β1 (TGF-β1) are added to replicate the fibrocartilage phase of bone. Quantitative RT-PCR analysis confirmed that this 3D fibrocartilage model enhances both osteogenesis and chondrogenesis, demonstrating its potential as a functional tissue model system [86].

9.4.6 Liver

Liver tissue engineering extensively employs primary hepatocytes and hepatocytes derived from stem cells. However, hepatocytes tend to lose their functional capacity quickly in culture. To address this issue, a novel approach has been developed using bioprinting technology to maintain long-term hepatocyte activity by forming hepatic cord-like structures, or "canaliculi." Rat hepatocytes cultivated in a collagen matrix exhibited canaliculi formation as early as day three, with functional markers such as the basolateral protein CD147 and the apical marker MRP2 confirming their activity [87]. Another strategy involves assessing hepatocyte function on various extracellular matrix (ECM)-based hydrogels. Primary human hepatocytes were cultured in hydrogels containing ECM components like Collagen Type I, hyaluronic acid (HA), and heparin-conjugated HA (HP) within hydrogel sandwiches for four weeks. These customized hydrogels supported enhanced hepatocyte metabolism and stable albumin and urea production, making them a promising platform for cell therapy, toxicology testing, and drug screening. A different approach for biofabricating a 3D liver model involves stacking rat and human hepatocytes with endothelial cells to form multilayered tissue structures [88]. This multilayered design shows promise as a liver mimic for drug testing and therapeutic applications. Additionally, a scaffold-free technique using acoustic nodes was developed to bioengineer 3D liver models. In a fluidic system, thousands of tissue spheroids can assemble into predefined structures within seconds. The architecture can be dynamically altered by adjusting wave frequencies, offering flexibility in design. Hepatocyte spheroids formed 3D liver models, and after six days in culture, bile canaliculi and gap junctions were detected through anti-MRP2 and anti-Connexin 32 immunostaining. This acoustic assembly method provides a fast, efficient way to create customizable 3D tissue models with precise geometric control and rapid pattern adjustment using vibration-guided spheroid assembly [89].

9.5 Bioprinting for Various Biomedical Applications

Recent advancements in cell manipulation and bioprinting technology have enabled various scientific applications, including the development of 3D models for drug testing and the cryoprinting of cells for biobanking purposes.

9.5.1 Drug Discovery

The development of in vitro tissue models holds significant potential for advancing drug discovery research. Among the many medical applications of 3D bioprinting, drug development stands out as an exciting and rapidly growing field, despite regulatory challenges that may delay progress in artificial organ technology. Recent technological advancements have accelerated drug design and discovery, but the lack of approved experimental platforms remains a challenge when using traditional 2D monolayer systems. In contrast, miniature 3D tissue models offer more accurate experimental platforms by closely mimicking the natural tissue environment [90], making them valuable for designing, discovering, and developing next-generation drugs. These 3D models promise to predict the success or failure of drugs during preclinical testing, providing a more accurate and cost-effective alternative to traditional in vitro or animal-based preclinical screening methods [91]. Additionally, 3D printing in drug development offers the benefits of customization and personalization of medications and medical devices, improving drug discovery efficiency while reducing preclinical trial costs. Various bioprinting techniques, such as cell spheroids, cell encapsulation, and microfluidic systems, have been utilized in drug screening studies. A recent innovation involves a droplet bioprinting method that produces sub-nanoliter droplets using an array-based drug screening platform, enabling multiplex protein assays based on CYP3A4 [92]. Another approach used a valve-based bioprinter to create a 3D lung model for drug evaluation, employing a layer-by-layer process to construct high-throughput screening architectures. By replicating complex cellular structures, 3D tissue models can enhance drug development and assessment while reducing the reliance on animal models in preclinical research.

9.5.2 Biopreservation

Traditional cryopreservation techniques, which rely on bulk cell storage, often lead to inadequate cooling and rewarming, causing cellular damage due to issues like ice crystal formation. Bioprinting offers a solution by converting large cell samples into micro- and nanoliter droplets, effectively addressing these challenges [93]. A recent innovation involved vitrifying red blood cells (RBCs) using a bioprinting method combined with advanced bio-inspired cryo-inks. This approach minimizes the need for high concentrations of cryoprotectants, as the bioprinter creates ultra-small droplets (< 0.15 nanoliters), significantly reducing adverse effects on RBCs [94]. The technique also provides ultrafast cooling and rewarming rates, preserving cells while preventing ice crystal formation. To avoid the toxicity of conventional cryoprotectants like glycerol and dimethyl sulfoxide, an ectoine-based bio-inspired cryo-ink was used as a safe, non-toxic alternative. Post-thaw, the biopreserved cells maintained their shape, functionality, and dynamics. This bio-inspired bioprinting method holds promise for regenerative and reproductive medicine, offering new possibilities for preserving cells such as stem cells, lymphocytes, and oocytes [95, 96].

9.6 Future Prospects and Challenges

This chapter highlights the guiding principles of 3D bioprinting in tissue fabrication, along with recent advancements and technological innovations. The rapid progress in additive manufacturing and automated printing systems demonstrates the promising potential to enhance scientific and engineering capabilities in addressing healthcare challenges. A significant milestone in 3D bioprinting is the ability to replicate and organize cellular microenvironments across molecular to macroscopic scales for tissue engineering and regenerative medicine [97]. Emerging 3D bioprinting technologies offer various strategies for fabricating tissue constructs, particularly for creating engineered 3D cell microenvironments to support artificial tissue development and deepen the understanding of cellular interactions and tissue formation. Cutting-edge technologies such as microfluidic systems, biopatterning, and layer-by-layer assembly have enabled the creation of micro-tissue constructs within scaffolds or scaffold-free environments [97]. However, several challenges remain. One of the most critical issues is vascularization, which limits tissue engineering and bioprinting efforts. Without adequate vascular networks, hypoxia, apoptosis, and rapid cell death can occur. Innovative solutions for developing vascular structures are urgently needed. While porous scaffolds have been used to facilitate vascularization, they do not fully resolve the issue due to limitations in cell and material diffusion [98]. Advances in bioprinting are expected to address these challenges by enabling the creation of interconnected, well-defined vascular networks during the manufacturing process. In addition to vascularization, ensuring mechanical strength and stability is essential in 3D tissue constructs, especially for regenerating hard tissues like bone and soft tissues like vascular grafts. Optimizing the elastic modulus of these constructs is crucial for their functionality. Another challenge lies in developing a fully integrated bioprinting system that encompasses both printing and post-printing processes, including in vitro culture and tissue maturation [99]. Overcoming these obstacles will pave the way for scaling up bioprinting technologies, leading to faster clinical solutions and advancements in medical implants. The integration of cells and biomaterials with microfluidic technologies has the potential to create specialized microenvironments for applications in cancer research, tissue engineering, and regenerative medicines [100].

References

1. Zhao S, Cong H, Pan T (2009) Direct projection on dry-film photoresist (DP2): do-it-yourself three-dimensional polymer microfluidics. Lab Chip 9:1128–1132
2. Malda J et al (2013) 25th anniversary article: engineering hydrogels for biofabrication. Adv Mater 25:5011–5028
3. Tasoglu S, Demirci U (2013) Bioprinting for stem cell research. Trends Biotechnol 31:10–19
4. Chanda A, Gupta S (2025) Healthcare entrepreneurship and management. Routledge, Taylor & Francis Group
5. Derby B (2012) Printing and prototyping of tissues and scaffolds. Science 338:921–926
6. Guillotin B, Guillemot F (2011) Cell patterning technologies for organotypic tissue fabrication. Trends Biotechnol 29:183–190
7. Zhang Y et al (2014) In vitro study of directly bioprinted perfusable vasculature conduits. Biomater Sci 3:134–143
8. Gupta S, Gupta V, Chanda A (2022) Biomechanical modeling of novel high expansion auxetic skin grafts. Int J Numer Method Biomed Eng 38:e3586
9. The 3D bioprinting revolution—Harvard Science Review. https://harvardsciencereview.org/2014/05/01/the-3d-bioprinting-revolution/
10. Williams JM et al (2005) Bone tissue engineering using polycaprolactone scaffolds fabricated via selective laser sintering. Biomaterials 26:4817–4827
11. Vaidya M (2015) Startups tout commercially 3D-printed tissue for drug screening. Nat Med 21:2
12. Singla R, Gupta S, Chanda A (2023) A computational fluid dynamics-based model for assessing rupture risk in cerebral arteries with varying aneurysm sizes. Math Comput Appl 28:90
13. Bose D, Gupta S, Chanda A (2025) Scalable direct manufacturing of a functional multipurpose wrist-hand orthosis using 3D printing. Ann 3D Print Med 17:100186
14. Bale SS et al (2014) In vitro platforms for evaluating liver toxicity. Exp Biol Med 239:1180–1191. https://doi.org/10.1177/1535370214531872
15. Gupta S, Singh G, Chanda A (2021) Prediction of diabetic foot ulcer progression: a computational study. Biomed Phys Eng Express 7:065020

16. Ellahi A, Gupta S, Bose D, Chanda A (2025) A high-fidelity biomechanical modeling framework for injury prediction during frontal car crash. Comput Methods Biomech Biomed Eng 28:13–24
17. Cui X, Gao G, Yonezawa T, Dai G (2014) Human cartilage tissue fabrication using three-dimensional inkjet printing technology. JoVE (J Vis Exp) e51294. https://doi.org/10.3791/51294
18. Kingsley DM, Dias AD, Chrisey DB, Corr DT (2013) Single-step laser-based fabrication and patterning of cell-encapsulated alginate microbeads. Biofabrication 5:045006
19. Ali M, Pages E, Ducom A, Fontaine A, Guillemot F (2014) Controlling laser-induced jet formation for bioprinting mesenchymal stem cells with high viability and high resolution. Biofabrication 6:045001
20. Hoch E, Tovar GEM, Borchers K (2014) Bioprinting of artificial blood vessels: current approaches towards a demanding goal. Eur J Cardio-Thoracic Surg 46:767–778
21. Moon SJ, Ceyhan E, Gurkan UA, Demirci U (2011) Statistical modeling of single target cell encapsulation. PLoS ONE 6:e21580
22. Moon S et al (2009) Layer by layer three-dimensional tissue epitaxy by cell-laden hydrogel droplets. Tissue Eng Part C Methods 16:157–166. https://home.liebertpub.com/tec
23. Kotlarz M, Ferreira AM, Gentile P, Russell SJ, Dalgarno K (2022) Droplet-based bioprinting enables the fabrication of cell–hydrogel–microfibre composite tissue precursors. Bio-Design Manuf 5:512–528
24. Ferris CJ, Gilmore KG, Wallace GG, In Het Panhuis M (2013) Biofabrication: an overview of the approaches used for printing of living cells. Appl Microbiol Biotechnol 97(10):4243–4258
25. Hribar KC, Soman P, Warner J, Chung P, Chen S (2013) Light-assisted direct-write of 3D functional biomaterials. Lab Chip 14:268–275
26. Minaeva ED et al (2023) Laser bioprinting with cell spheroids: accurate and gentle. Micromachines 14:1152
27. Gruene M et al (2011) Laser printing of stem cells for biofabrication of scaffold-free autologous grafts. Tissue Eng Part C Methods 17:79–87
28. Koch L et al (2009) Laser printing of skin cells and human stem cells. Tissue Eng Part C Methods 16:847–854. https://home.liebertpub.com/tec
29. Jones N (2012) Science in three dimensions: the print revolution. Nature 487:22–23
30. Yadav P et al (2025) Gelatin multiwalled carbon nanotube composite 3D printed semi biological mesh for abdominal hernia treatment. Chem Asian J20:e202401136
31. Chhikara K, Sidhu SS, Gupta S, Saharawat S, Kataria C, Chanda A (2023) Development and effectiveness testing of a novel 3D-printed multi-material orthosis in nurses with plantar foot pain. Prosthesis 5:73–87
32. Rothschild BM et al (2023) Design, manufacturing, and trial of a 3D printed customized finger splint for patients with rheumatoid arthritis. Rheumato 3:51–62
33. Cohen DL, Lipton JI, Bonassar LJ, Lipson H (2010) Additive manufacturing for in situ repair of osteochondral defects. Biofabrication 2
34. Sonaye SY, Ertugral EG, Kothapalli CR, Sikder P (2022) Extrusion 3D (Bio)Printing of alginate-gelatin-based composite scaffolds for skeletal muscle tissue engineering. Materials 15:7945
35. Yadav P, Kamboj M, Das B (2024) Application of nanotechnology in antimicrobial coating on surgical instruments. Appl Nanotechnol Biomed Eng 150–168. https://doi.org/10.1201/9781003432661-9
36. Zhang X et al (2012) Nanoliter droplet vitrification for oocyte cryopreservation. Nanomedicine 7:553–564
37. Singh G, Chanda A (2024) Development and biomechanical testing of artificial surrogates for vaginal tissue. Adv Mater Process Technol. https://doi.org/10.1080/2374068X.2023.2198837
38. Chanda A (2018) Biomechanical modeling of human skin tissue surrogates. Biomimetics 3:18

39. El Assal R et al (2014) Bio-inspired cryo-ink preserves red blood cell phenotype and function during nanoliter vitrification. Adv Mater 26:5815–5822
40. Enam S, Jin S (2015) Substrates for clinical applicability of stem cells. World J Stem Cells 7:243
41. Pearce ME, Melanko JB, Salem AK (2007) Multifunctional nanorods for biomedical applications. Pharm Res 24:2335–2352
42. Foss C, Merzari E, Migliaresi C, Motta A (2013) Silk fibroin/hyaluronic acid 3D matrices for cartilage tissue engineering. Biomacromol 14:38–47
43. Ural E, Kesenci K, Fambri L, Migliaresi C, Piskin E (2000) Poly(d,l-cactide/ε-caprolactone)/hydroxyapatite composites. Biomaterials 21:2147–2154
44. Gurkan UA, Tasoglu S, Kavaz D, Demirel MC, Demirci U (2012) Emerging technologies for assembly of microscale hydrogels. Adv Healthc Mater 1:149–158
45. Guvendiren M, Burdick JA (2013) Engineering synthetic hydrogel microenvironments to instruct stem cells. Curr Opin Biotechnol 24:841–846
46. Hunt NC, Grover LM (2010) Cell encapsulation using biopolymer gels for regenerative medicine. Biotechnol Lett 32:733–742
47. Poldervaart MT et al (2014) Prolonged presence of VEGF promotes vascularization in 3D bioprinted scaffolds with defined architecture. J Control Release 184:58–66
48. Bölgen N, Vargel I, Korkusuz P, Menceloğlu YZ, Pişkin E (2007) In vivo performance of antibiotic embedded electrospun PCL membranes for prevention of abdominal adhesions. J Biomed Mater Res B Appl Biomater 81:530–543
49. Watson BM et al (2015) Biodegradable, phosphate-containing, dual-gelling macromers for cellular delivery in bone tissue engineering. Biomaterials 67:286–296
50. Leung GKK, Wang YC, Wu W (2012) Peptide nanofiber scaffold for brain tissue reconstruction. Methods Enzymol 508:177–190
51. Chanda A, Chatterjee S, Gupta V (2020) Soft composite based hyperelastic model for anisotropic tissue characterization. J Compos Mater 54:4525–4534
52. Verma S, Singh G, Chanda A (2023) A novel finite element model for the study of harmful vibrations on the aging spine. Computation 11:93
53. Bourgine PE et al (2014) Osteoinductivity of engineered cartilaginous templates devitalized by inducible apoptosis. Proc Natl Acad Sci U S A 111:17426–17431
54. Puppi D et al (2012) Additive manufacturing of wet-spun polymeric scaffolds for bone tissue engineering. Biomed Microdevices 14:1115–1127
55. Verma S, Singh G, Chanda A (2024) Development of a computational framework for determination of detrimental vibrations on the human spine segments. Multiscale Sci Eng 61(6):48–56
56. Verma S, Chanda A (2024) State-of-the-art of finite element modelling of the human spine to study the impact of vibrations: a review. Int J Comput Methods Eng Sci Mech25:225–247
57. Singh G, Chanda A (2024) Liver tissue surrogates: development and biomechanical characterization. Spectr Mech Eng Oper Res 1:121–130
58. Chanda A, Singh G (2024) Gallbladder tissue simulants, pp 113–123. https://doi.org/10.1007/978-981-97-3060-5_11
59. Chanda A, Singh G (2024) Heart tissue simulants, pp 71–82. https://doi.org/10.1007/978-981-97-3060-5_7
60. Chanda A, Singh G (2024) Simulants for arteries, pp 125–136. https://doi.org/10.1007/978-981-97-3060-5_12
61. Singh G, Chanda A (2021) Mechanical properties of whole-body soft human tissues: a review. Biomed Mater 16:062004
62. Chanda A, Singh G (2024) Muscle tissue simulants, pp 37–49. https://doi.org/10.1007/978-981-97-3060-5_4
63. Chanda A, Singh G (2024) Lung tissue simulants, pp 59–70. https://doi.org/10.1007/978-981-97-3060-5_6
64. Chanda A, Singh G (2024) Stomach tissue simulants, pp 103–112. https://doi.org/10.1007/978-981-97-3060-5_10

65. Chanda A, Singh G (2024) Breast tissue simulants, pp 83–91. https://doi.org/10.1007/978-981-97-3060-5_8
66. Mironov V et al (2009) Organ printing: tissue spheroids as building blocks. Biomaterials 30:2164–2174
67. Sohn SH, Kim TH, Kim TS, Min TJ, Lee JH, Yoo SM, Kim JW, Lee JE, Kim C, Park S-H, Jo WM (2021) Evaluation of 3D templated synthetic vascular graft compared with standard graft in a rat model: potential use as an artificial vascular graft in cardiovascular disease. Materials 14(5):1239
68. Lee VK et al (2014) Creating perfused functional vascular channels using 3D bio-printing technology. Biomaterials 35:8092–8102
69. Afazal M, Afreen S, Chanda A (2023) Computational modelling and analysis of hard tissue behavior around 0.5 mm and 0.85 mm platform switched abutment using 3D finite element analysis. Forces Mech 13:100243
70. Chanda A, Unnikrishnan V, Flynn Z, Lackey K (2017) Experimental study on tissue phantoms to understand the effect of injury and suturing on human skin mechanical properties. Proc Inst Mech Eng Part H J Eng Med 231:80–91
71. Skardal A et al (2012) Bioprinted amniotic fluid-derived stem cells accelerate healing of large skin wounds. Stem Cells Transl Med 1:792–802
72. Biofidelic skin simulant (2018)
73. Chanda A, Singh G (2024) Skin tissue simulants, pp 23–36. https://doi.org/10.1007/978-981-97-3060-5_3
74. Chanda A, Callaway C (2018) Tissue anisotropy modeling using soft composite materials. Appl Bionics Biomech 2018:4838157
75. Singh G, Gupta V, Chanda A (2022) Artificial skin with varying biomechanical properties. Mater Today Proc 62:3162–3166
76. Chanda A (2018) Customized human skin simulants. https://doi.org/10.31219/OSF.IO/S74N5
77. Nath Yadav P, Singh G, Chanda A (2022) Biomechanical modeling of cerebral aneurysm. Mater Today Proc 62:3295–3300
78. Chanda A, Singh G (2024) Brain tissue simulants, pp 51–58. https://doi.org/10.1007/978-981-97-3060-5_5
79. Chanda A, Unnikrishnan V (2016) Human tissue simulants for study of traumatic brain injury (TBI). Proceedings of the American society for composites 2016—thirty-first technical conference
80. Singh G, Chanda A (2023) Development and mechanical characterization of artificial surrogates for brain tissues. Biomed Eng Adv 5:100084
81. Chanda A, Callaway C, Clifton C, Unnikrishnan V (2018) Biofidelic human brain tissue surrogates. Mech Adv Mater Struct 25:1335–1341
82. Lorber B, Hsiao WK, Hutchings IM, Martin KR (2014) Adult rat retinal ganglion cells and glia can be printed by piezoelectric inkjet printing. Biofabrication 6
83. Fedorovich NE, Haverslag RT, Dhert WJA, Alblas J (2010) The role of endothelial progenitor cells in prevascularized bone tissue engineering: development of heterogeneous constructs. Tissue Eng Part A 16:2355–2367
84. Pensak MJ, Lieberman JR (2013) Gene therapy for bone regeneration. Curr Pharm Des 19:3466–3473
85. Loozen LD, Wegman F, Öner FC, Dhert WJA, Alblas J (2013) Porous bioprinted constructs in BMP-2 non-viral gene therapy for bone tissue engineering. J Mater Chem B 1:6619–6626
86. Si-Tayeb K et al (2010) Highly efficient generation of human hepatocyte-like cells from induced pluripotent stem cells. Hepatology 51:297–305
87. Casado JG et al (2014) Mesenchymal stem cell-coated sutures enhance collagen depositions in sutured tissues. Wound Repair Regen 22:256–264
88. Chang R, Emami K, Wu H, Sun W (2010) Biofabrication of a three-dimensional liver micro-organ as an in vitro drug metabolism model. Biofabrication 2
89. Chanda A, Singh G (2024) Liver tissue simulants, pp 93–101. https://doi.org/10.1007/978-981-97-3060-5_9

90. Xiong A et al (2008) Isolation of human fetal liver progenitors and their enhanced proliferation by three-dimensional coculture with endothelial cells. Tissue Eng Part A 14:995
91. Charoen KM, Fallica B, Colson YL, Zaman MH, Grinstaff MW (2014) Embedded multicellular spheroids as a biomimetic 3D cancer model for evaluating drug and drug-device combinations. Biomaterials 35:2264–2271
92. Arrabito G, Galati C, Castellano S, Pignataro B (2012) Luminometric sub-nanoliter droplet-to-droplet array (LUMDA) and its application to drug screening by phase I metabolism enzymes. Lab Chip 13:68–72
93. Guven S et al (2015) Functional maintenance of differentiated embryoid bodies in microfluidic systems: a platform for personalized medicine. Stem Cells Transl Med 4:261–268
94. Kline M, Dreyer M, Gyring P, Lifson M, El Assal R (2015) 60. Innovative cryoprotectants for tissue and organ preservation. Cryobiology 71:180
95. Zhang X, Catalano PN, Gurkan UA, Khimji I, Demirci U (2011) Emerging technologies in medical applications of minimum volume vitrification. Nanomedicine (London) 6:1115
96. Gupta V, Singh G, Chanda A (2023) Development of hierarchical auxetic skin graft simulants with high expansion potential. Biomed Eng Adv 5:100087
97. Dado D, Levenberg S (2009) Cell-scaffold mechanical interplay within engineered tissue. Semin Cell Dev Biol 20:656–664
98. Mironov V, Boland T, Trusk T, Forgacs G, Markwald RR (2003) Organ printing: computer-aided jet-based 3D tissue engineering. Trends Biotechnol 21:157–161
99. Prestwich GD (2011) Hyaluronic acid-based clinical biomaterials derived for cell and molecule delivery in regenerative medicine. J Control Release 155:193–199
100. Gurkan UA et al (2011) Controlled viable release of selectively captured label-free cells in microchannels. Lab Chip 11:3979–3989

GPSR Compliance
The European Union's (EU) General Product Safety Regulation (GPSR) is a set of rules that requires consumer products to be safe and our obligations to ensure this.

If you have any concerns about our products, you can contact us on

ProductSafety@springernature.com

In case Publisher is established outside the EU, the EU authorized representative is:

Springer Nature Customer Service Center GmbH
Europaplatz 3
69115 Heidelberg, Germany

www.ingramcontent.com/pod-product-compliance
Ingram Content Group UK Ltd.
Pitfield, Milton Keynes, MK11 3LW, UK
UKHW020632260926
475829UK00003BA/52

* 9 7 8 9 8 1 9 2 1 3 0 6 1 *